# the
# wellness
# trap

# the
# wellness
# trap

### Break Free
### from
### DIET CULTURE,
### DISINFORMATION,
### and DUBIOUS
### DIAGNOSES—and Find
### Your True Well-Being

## Christy Harrison, MPH, RD

Little, Brown Spark
New York Boston London

Hachette Book Group supports the right to free expression and the value of copyright. The purpose of copyright is to encourage writers and artists to produce the creative works that enrich our culture.

The scanning, uploading, and distribution of this book without permission is a theft of the author's intellectual property. If you would like permission to use material from the book (other than for review purposes), please contact permissions@hbgusa.com. Thank you for your support of the author's rights.

Little, Brown Spark
Hachette Book Group
1290 Avenue of the Americas, New York, NY 10104
littlebrownspark.com

First Edition: April 2023

Little, Brown Spark is an imprint of Little, Brown and Company, a division of Hachette Book Group, Inc. The Little, Brown Spark name and logo are trademarks of Hachette Book Group, Inc.

The publisher is not responsible for websites (or their content) that are not owned by the publisher.

The Hachette Speakers Bureau provides a wide range of authors for speaking events. To find out more, go to hachettespeakersbureau.com or email HachetteSpeakers@hbgusa.com.

LCCN is available at the Library of Congress

Printing 1, 2023

ISBN 978-0-316-31560-9

LSC-C

Printed in the United States of America

*For my daughter*

# Table of Contents

# the
# wellness
# trap

# Introduction

Between the ages of twenty-one and twenty-two, I was diagnosed with three chronic conditions common among women: Hashimoto's thyroiditis, an autoimmune disease that causes the thyroid to attack itself, causing hypothyroidism or low thyroid levels; gastroesophageal reflux disease (GERD), a more severe and persistent form of acid reflux; and polycystic ovarian syndrome (PCOS), a condition that causes hormonal imbalances and (in some cases) small cysts on the ovaries. That last one turned out to be a misdiagnosis, but in the years that followed I developed a laundry list of other conditions, including irritable bowel syndrome (IBS), immune thrombocytopenia (ITP), eczema, a hiatal hernia, plantar fasciitis, chronic tendinitis in my left wrist, multiple environmental allergies, and a binocular vision disorder that caused occasional migraines and phobias of heights and highway driving. Psychotherapists also diagnosed me with generalized anxiety disorder, panic disorder with agoraphobia, and post-traumatic stress disorder (PTSD) related to events in my childhood and beyond, including an emotionally abusive relationship in my early twenties.

Ironically, that was the time in my life when I was most obsessed with wellness—which in my mind was synonymous with thinness and "perfect" eating. It was the early days of the Internet, before social media dumped an onslaught of wellness misinformation into the mainstream, so I got mine from message boards devoted to specific conditions (including celiac disease, which for a time I was convinced I had). While for some people a fixation on wellness starts precisely because they're having health problems, in hindsight I can see that for me it was the pursuit of wellness *itself* that triggered at least some of my conditions: digestive issues because I was caught up in a restrict-binge cycle with food (which wreaks havoc on the GI tract), plantar fasciitis because I was overexercising, and the PCOS misdiagnosis because I wasn't eating enough to get my period— a condition called hypothalamic amenorrhea, which can cause many of the symptoms of PCOS. Trauma also may have played a role, as it does for many people with chronic illness: PTSD has been shown to be associated with hypothyroidism,[1] IBS,[2] and eczema,[3] among other disorders.

Now, nearly two decades later, my relationship with food and my body is better than ever, and I do my best to get my health advice from trusted sources and block out dubious ones—which are more prolific and harmful than ever before, as we'll discuss. I still have these conditions, and occasionally they flare up and interfere with my life, as they did during my pregnancy and childbirth. I'm one of 60 percent of adults in the US with a chronic disease, and one of the 40 percent with two or more.[4] Yet for the most part, I feel and function as well as most people I know without chronic illnesses.

Not everyone is as fortunate, and social factors have a lot to do with why: exposure to persistent racial discrimination and lower socioeconomic status have been shown to predict both a greater number of chronic illnesses[5] and poorer access to quality healthcare for them.[6] These disparities were only magnified by the COVID-19 pandemic, which disproportionately affected people of color and those of lower socioeconomic status, especially early on. (According to an analysis by *The Washington Post*, in the fall of 2021 COVID death rates among white Americans began to surpass those among Black Americans—not because Black people were facing fewer barriers to care, but because so many white people were going unvaccinated and unmasked for ideological reasons.[7]) A study conducted in 2020 of more than thirty-one hundred U.S. counties found that both COVID case rates and death rates were significantly higher in counties with larger Black populations and higher percentages of adults who hadn't graduated high school; those with larger Hispanic populations also had significantly higher case rates (though the difference in death rates was not significant once confounding factors were controlled for).[8] As an April 2020 article headline in *The Cut* asked, "In a pandemic, is 'wellness' just being well-off? Maybe there isn't really a difference anymore."

That raises the question: What is wellness, really? It's typically defined as a practice of seeking to prevent illness and prolong life, as opposed to simply treating diseases (although people with diseases make up a significant part of the wellness market), with a clear emphasis on individual choice and responsibility. It's only natural when you're ill (whether acutely or chronically) to want to feel better, to not be in pain. But that's not what wellness means in this current culture; wellness is not simply the opposite of illness. The Global Wellness Institute (GWI), a nonprofit research and advocacy group whose mission is "to empower wellness worldwide," says that "wellness is not a passive or static state but rather an 'active pursuit' that is associated with intentions, choices, and actions as we work toward an optimal state of health and wellbeing."[9] While the GWI nods to the role of "the physical, social and cultural environments in which we live," ultimately they paint the path to wellness as "an active process of being aware and making choices that lead toward an outcome of optimal holistic health and wellbeing."

In other words, wellness is defined by the things you *do*. And doing those things typically requires a fair amount of economic privilege: As a 2021 *New Yorker* article humorously put it, "wellness...encompasses a broad range of activities, including juice cleansing, Transcendental Meditation, snail-serum application, buying a Peloton, napping, switching to oat milk, switching to charcoal water, Kegel exercises, sitz baths, citrus diets, maintaining ketosis, HIIT [high-intensity interval training] workouts, halotherapy, aromatherapy, talk therapy, past-life regression therapy, microdosing LSD, megadosing CBD, intuitive fasting, avoiding blue light, seeking out red light, reflexology, cathartic-breathing techniques, the Alexander Technique, sensory deprivation, forest bathing, and gargling with Himalayan salt."[10]

Wellness *culture* is the belief system that underlies all these pursuits. It's a set of values that equates wellness with moral goodness and posits certain behaviors—and a certain type of body—as the path to achieving that supposed rectitude. Wellness culture overlaps with diet culture, which I described in my first book, *Anti-Diet*, as a system of beliefs that equates thinness, muscularity, and particular body shapes with health and moral virtue; promotes weight loss and body reshaping as a means of attaining higher status; demonizes certain foods and food groups while elevating others; and oppresses people who don't match its supposed picture of health. Wellness culture more or less incorporates these values wholesale from diet culture, but it also adds several other major tenets of its own: denigrating conventional medicine and idolizing alternative, "integrative," "natural," and "holistic" approaches to healing, with a particular reverence for methods perceived as "ancient" and non-Western (even if those characterizations aren't always accurate); stressing the importance of the individual's ability to pick and choose which wellness practices to adopt, in a way that often results in taking healing modalities out of context and creating cultural appropriation and fetishization; lionizing individual choices in general, downplaying or outright ignoring the social determinants of health that have a far greater impact on people's well-being than individual behaviors; and giving anecdotes and social media testimonials more weight than sound scientific evidence, enabling the spread of mis- and disinformation.

In many ways, wellness is the rich person's version of health.

Both concepts are often exclusionary, but wellness has an added layer of elitism to it, because it's about the relentless *pursuit* of the apex of health, in a way that only people who are rich in both time and money can truly afford. "To seek out healing near constantly when you don't have a profound illness is arguably a hobby, a pastime," says comedian Jacqueline Novak in the first episode of the Poog podcast, a show co-hosted by Novak and comedian Kate Berlant that sends up wellness culture (Poog is *goop*, the name of Gwyneth Paltrow's brand, spelled backwards) while also being very much a part of it.[11] As we'll discuss in the following chapters, wellness is a hobby that can have disastrous consequences for its participants, even as it enriches the industry. You might say that wellness is to true well-being what social media is to human connection: an ongoing attempt to attain the pinnacle of the thing, which only sometimes succeeds and more often takes people further from their objectives, to the tune of billions of dollars per year.

In the case of wellness, it's actually trillions: The worldwide wellness market was worth $4.4 trillion in 2020, according to the GWI, which tracks wellness-industry growth.[12] (A 2021 estimate by the consulting firm McKinsey & Company puts it at a more modest $1.5 trillion, but that includes fewer segments under the umbrella of wellness.[13]) The GWI's breakdown includes a $413 billion market for "traditional and complementary medicine," a $375 billion market for "public health, prevention, and personalized medicine," a $738 billion market for physical activity, and a staggering $955 billion market for personal care and beauty, which includes anti-aging treatments. It also includes a $121 billion market for an emerging category called mental wellness, which according to the GWI is distinct from traditional mental health in that it's possible to have a diagnosed mental illness but still be in a state of positive mental wellness, and it's also possible *not* to be "'mentally well' or thriving" even if you *don't* have a diagnosed mental illness. The mental-wellness market includes a wide array of things that *goop* (or Poog) has probably covered: mind-body practices such as yoga, tai chi, qigong, and breathwork (ancient traditions with their own cultural significance outside of Western wellness culture, which have become commodified by that culture); sensory products and experiences like massage, reiki, weighted blankets, aromatherapy, and sound therapy; "brain-boosting nutraceuticals and botanicals" such as "natural" supplements, herbs, traditional remedies, and cannabis derivatives like CBD; self-help and personal development groups, "gurus," and books; sleep products and technologies like sleep accessories, smart bedding, sleep retreats, and wearables to track your sleep; meditation and mindfulness practices; and classes, retreats, and apps.[14] As GWI's vice president of research said in 2020, although the wellness industry saw some contraction during COVID-19, "at the big-picture, long-term level, the case for the wellness concept and wellness markets post-pandemic looks very bullish."[15]

Perhaps the most culturally impactful segment of the global wellness industry, if not the most lucrative, is the $946 billion global market for "healthy eating," nutrition, and weight loss. For many people, wellness is synonymous with food and body size. As I described in *Anti-Diet*, diet culture has morphed and shape-shifted in the twenty-first century in order to stay relevant to a new generation who are more likely to eschew traditional diets in favor of "wellness." This new face of diet culture is what I call the *wellness diet*, which pretends to be all about achieving the pinnacle of health but is actually grounded in the same harmful value system that had people swallowing tapeworms in the early 1900s and fat-free everything in the 1980s and '90s in a largely futile quest for thinness. Indeed, somewhere north of 90 percent of weight-loss efforts fail after more than a year or two, and as many as two-thirds of people who embark on them end up gaining back more than they lost.[16] In *The Wellness Trap*, we'll discuss how wellness culture both overlaps with diet culture and propounds its own unique set of harmful beliefs, endorses dangerous practices, and partners with questionable industries. Elimination diets and "clean eating" are often people's first stop on the train to all kinds of other unproven wellness practices and false diagnoses, as you'll see in the following chapters.

Wellness misinformation doesn't affect everyone equally. It's especially concerning when it targets women, people of color, and marginalized people who health institutions have failed in countless ways over the course of centuries. It's only natural that those who've been let down by conventional medicine would want to explore other options. Unfortunately, though, some of those alternatives are more destructive than the treatments they seek to replace or the diseases they intend to prevent or cure. Some purveyors of wellness misinformation have been misled themselves, while others are unscrupulous, sophisticated actors spreading misinformation to capitalize on people's confusion and pain. (The latter group are better characterized as peddlers of *disinformation*—false information spread deliberately with the intent to deceive.) The wellness world is rife with conspiracy theories that are making their purveyors millions while threatening public health, as Chapters 4 and 5 will explore. Wellness culture is also replete with scams, schemes, and snake oil, as we'll discuss in Chapter 7.

To be clear, this book isn't about shaming anyone for falling into these traps. We're all just doing the best we can to take care of ourselves, but the system is set up to take advantage of our desire for self-care and security. The world can be a scary place, and wellness culture promises to make it safer by reducing your risks—so it's no wonder so many people are drawn to it. Far be it from me to take away something that makes you feel better. Life is hard, and we need all the help we can get—especially those of us with chronic illnesses, disabilities, and other forms of marginalization. It's only human to look for ways to cope, and it's a sign of our resilience that we try.

Not only that, but for some people wellness culture can even be fun. I get it: many of the products are luxurious and beautiful, and some of the practices are ritualistic in a way that can be comforting and make you feel connected to a community. It also can be delicious to get a glimpse of an "aspirational lifestyle," even if it's one you'll never be able to afford. I've seen wellness-retreat websites, and bottles of *goop* serums on friends' bathroom shelves, and felt a pang of longing for the life they represent. I've swooned over the scent of essential oils and blissed out at breathwork classes. Even as a critic of wellness culture, I'm not immune to its charms, and I'm not trying to kill anyone's joy here. If you like wellness and it's not hurting you, by all means do your thing.

Yet as I and many of the people you'll meet in these pages can attest, sometimes the things we think are helping us feel better are actually making matters worse. Sometimes the products and practices that once seemed to bring us relief—maybe even just the mental relief of believing we'd found a solution—become a source of greater harm. I wrote this book for anyone who's been through that experience, and for anyone who has a nagging feeling that wellness culture might be problematic, despite liking some of what it has to offer.

I often get questions from clients and readers along the lines of: "My functional-medicine doctor (or chiropractor/acupuncturist/naturopath) told me I need to eliminate X, Y, and Z foods in order to reverse my autoimmune disease (or prevent diabetes, or reduce inflammation), but it's ruining my relationship with food. How do I make peace with food while also following this diet?" Initially I thought perhaps there was some benefit to those diets, but through my research I've come to realize that more often than not, there's little to no good evidence behind them—and in fact they can actively undermine many people's well-being. I've found that the same is true for numerous herbal and dietary supplements, alternative-medicine practices, and other wellness-culture products and interventions.

That said, I do think there are some aspects of wellness culture that are useful and some practices that are evidence based. For example, systematic reviews of randomized controlled trials comparing post-traumatic stress interventions that included yoga and those that did not have found that the former lead to significantly lower physiological stress levels and improvement in PTSD symptoms, among other potential benefits.[17] Similar studies of mindfulness meditation have found evidence that it helps reduce anxiety, depression, and pain.[18] Granted, science isn't infallible, and there are undoubtedly some wellness-culture interventions that haven't made it into scientific studies yet (though fewer than you might think, as we'll discuss). There are also practices embedded within entire cultural worldviews that would be difficult, if not impossible, to study scientifically; for example, certain Indigenous healing traditions might be helpful for members of that community, but it would be culturally appropriative and damaging to try to transport those practices to another context (though that certainly doesn't stop some researchers from doing it). Such instances notwithstanding, I've found that for most popular products and practices in wellness culture, science is still the best method available for determining whether they have any real benefits beyond the placebo effect. Good science allows us to distinguish between useful interventions and ineffective or harmful ones. And science (or pseudoscience) is the language that wellness-culture proponents often use to try to sell their products and programs, so it's important to be able to critically assess what the scientific evidence really says. I'll be doing that throughout the book, and in later chapters I'll offer some thoughts on how to do it yourself.

This book will challenge a lot of beliefs about wellness that many people have internalized, so I know it's likely to elicit some feelings of resistance. I used to experience such resistance myself. If that's what happens for you, I'd invite you to stay curious, keep an open mind, and try to analyze, compassionately and nonjudgmentally, any cognitive dissonance that arises. When you've been told for years or decades that you need to do certain things in order to take care of your health, it's completely understandable to feel defensive when someone comes along challenging those beliefs.

That might go double when it's someone who looks like me — a white, relatively thin, relatively able-bodied (albeit chronically ill, formerly eating-disordered) cisgender woman, with all the unearned advantages that those identities afford me in our society. I understand that response, and I know my perspective has limitations, as everyone's does. With that awareness, I've strived to incorporate interviews with and citations by many people from more marginalized backgrounds than mine. I also reference as much research as possible that was conducted in large, diverse populations.

As in my first book, I don't include weight or calorie numbers because of their potential to trigger disordered behaviors in vulnerable people, and I make every effort to avoid stigmatizing language (e.g., using terms such as "larger-bodied" or "higher-weight" instead of clinical terminology that many people find derogatory). Still, in critiquing the anti-fat bias, healthism, and ableism inherent in contemporary wellness culture and its historical origins, I do sometimes quote sources that exemplify these forms of stigma. Similarly, the book contains some descriptions of harmful wellness-culture practices, though I do my best not to go into too much detail about them. There are also brief mentions of suicide and infant loss, and more in-depth discussions of cancer, chronic illnesses, eating disorders, conspiracy theories, racism and misogyny in medicine, and various forms of trauma. Please consider this a content warning for the pages ahead. (If you are in crisis, call or text 988 in the U.S., or visit befrienders.org.)

Given that people who critique alternative medicine and wellness culture are often painted as shills for "Big Pharma" and/or "Big Food," it might be helpful to mention my bona fides: I never have and never will accept any money from the pharmaceutical industry or major food manufacturers (though I did work at a couple of independent restaurants and cafes in the past, and I once ran an ad for a small tea company on my podcast *Food Psych*). No special-interest group is paying me to say any of the things I write in these pages (which would be illegal under the terms of my book contract). I'm no fan of pharmaceutical companies or many aspects of the medical industry, especially for their role in promoting diet culture and anti-fat bias, and I've been critical of many weight-loss studies funded by drug makers. But I also can't write off pharmaceuticals entirely, because I wouldn't be able to function without the thyroid medication that I take every day for my Hashimoto's disease, and my attempts to "fix it with food" only resulted in deeply disordered eating that took me years to dig my way out of. Similarly, I'm no apologist for food companies that promote diet culture and/or exploit their workers and the environment, yet I've also come to see just how mentally damaging—not to mention racist and classist—it can be to demonize "processed" foods and the food industry at large. I also can't deny that I'm a member of the wellness industry (if a reluctant one), as both a dietitian who specializes in intuitive eating and a journalist covering food, nutrition, and health. And I've personally found great relief in certain healing modalities that are very much a part of wellness culture, including yoga, meditation, and somatic psychotherapy.

If I'm skeptical of certain aspects of wellness culture, it's because of what I've learned through years of research and professional and personal experience, which I aim to at least begin to articulate in this book. In particular, both my own history and my work as a dietitian have shown me that wellness culture is creating rampant disordered eating. I've seen far too many clients driven to extremely restrictive and obsessive relationships with food by alternative-medicine providers and social media wellness influencers. And from dieting it can be a slippery slope to other dangerous practices. People often think of complementary and alternative treatments as harmless, or at least much less risky than conventional medicine, but in my experience that's definitely not the case. "Natural" therapies can have side effects that rival and even exceed those of standard medical care, and in many instances they don't work at all. Misdiagnoses from wellness practitioners (and the Internet) can prevent people from receiving accurate labels for their illnesses and getting the competent care they deserve. And in recent years it's also become clear that wellness culture can lead down rabbit holes of mis- and disinformation that threaten not just public health but society itself, as we'll discuss in Chapters 4 and 5.

What I'm hoping to do in *The Wellness Trap*, more than anything, is to offer a model for thinking critically about the wellness information you encounter, in order to help you avoid falling prey to toxic ideas about toxins, noxious beliefs about inoculations, and all the other dubious diagnoses and spurious cures proliferating every day. We'll start by analyzing how wellness culture became entangled with diet culture, and how wellness diets can lead to other problematic practices. We'll look at some of the pernicious effects of the supplement industry, the often misguided, if not injurious, "wellness" approach to mental health and trauma, and the rampant cultural appropriation that underlies many popular corners of wellness culture. Then we'll talk through how social media algorithms are leading to a proliferation of wellness mis- and disinformation that's threatening both individual and public health. Finally, we'll explore what it would look like to move from the current manifestation of wellness culture to a society that promotes true well-being for all its members.

# CHAPTER 1

# Wellness and Diet Culture

Maxine Ali, now a researcher studying women's relationships with wellness culture, was caught up in it herself in 2013, just as she was getting ready to go off to college. She'd been diagnosed with ulcerative colitis, a type of inflammatory bowel disease, at the age of twelve, so by the time she turned eighteen she'd been chronically ill for years. She'd struggled with restrictive eating and body-image issues for just as long, having turned to dieting to try to lose the weight she'd gained on medication for colitis. As a teenager growing up in a small rural town about an hour outside London, she'd tried a few wellness-y things, including a gluten-free, dairy-free diet and homeopathic treatments, which her mother had hoped would help ease her symptoms without the side effects of medication. But it wasn't until Ali started following early-Instagram wellness influencers that she really got hooked into wellness culture. "There were all these beautiful people on social media saying how they'd cured themselves of X, Y, and Z because they'd been eating a 'clean' diet, they'd been cutting out dairy, and gluten, and sugar, and all of this other stuff," she says. Some of these influencers said they'd healed from chronic illnesses similar to the one Ali had. Others claimed to have overcome terminal cancer through food and alternative medicine alone. For someone who was sick of being sick—and of thinking she *looked* sick—the world of wellness culture and its glowing, young, conventionally attractive representatives proved irresistibly seductive.

Soon she joined their ranks by starting a wellness blog, doing an internship at a UK women's fitness magazine, and eventually becoming a digital editor at a wellness brand. At first she loved working in wellness media, but looking back she now sees how harmful it really was. "It was a culture of disordered eating," she says. At the fitness magazine, the office was filled with women on perpetual diets, who measured everything they ate and did regular juice cleanses. The same was true of the wellness brand, where she says there was a toxic culture of over-exercise and overwork, and pressure to be (or at least look like) "the epitome of health." As a mixed-race woman, Ali was one of the only people of color in the workplace. She was simultaneously asked to help the company bring more diversity to its wellness coverage and not given any power to make that happen.

Being in those environments dramatically worsened her disordered eating. It also made her feel justified in her restrictive behaviors, which, looking back, she now sees only worsened her colitis. "It kind of legitimized what I was doing as healthy, because when you're working in an industry that is supposed to be disseminating health information and you see this kind of behavior, you think, 'well, this must be what health looks like.'"

It was more than just the promise of better health that ensnared her in the wellness trap, though—it was the promise of a more successful career, a more exciting social life, and a better existence all around. The editors she worked with "were living these incredibly glamorous lives, going to all of these high-end boutique fitness studios and getting all these wellness treatments," she says. They were portraying an "aspirational lifestyle" that didn't just look like surviving and getting by while managing a chronic illness—it looked like thriving. It looked like fun. "That's the way wellness is painted," Ali says. "It's not just about the health. It's about everything that comes with it."

"Everything that comes with it" is in many ways what drives

people toward wellness culture. Whether you're struggling with chronic health conditions or not, striving toward a mythical ideal of wellness is held out as the secret to the happiness and security that people understandably seek, especially in an uncertain world. We're told that preventing illness is the holy grail, the key to the good life—and that if we do happen to get sick, managing our illnesses in the "right" way, the "natural" way, through diet and exercise, will help us feel just as good as if we'd never been sick in the first place. Wellness brands and entrepreneurs are right there to sell us those supposedly correct and natural methods, which are hopelessly out of reach for millions of people—though often we don't realize it at the time.

That certainly was the case for me. Like Ali, when I was a young journalist grappling with my own health issues, I got swept up in a vision of wellness that relied heavily on restrictive eating. I spent hours each day thinking about, preparing, and purchasing food that was as "clean" and "whole" as possible, then second-guessing my choices and often getting lost in research about the purported harms and benefits of different ingredients. I believed that if I could just crack the code on how to "eat right," I could send my chronic diseases into remission and prevent all future health problems (and get the body of a willowy yoga model in the process, though I didn't say that part out loud).

The wellness ideal was unattainable and damaging to my well-being, and I unwittingly transmitted it—via a lot of proselytizing about local, "whole," "real" food—to my readers. It was the early 2000s, and wellness culture was nowhere near the well-oiled (essential-oiled?) machine it's become in the age of social media, but already its ethos of food- and weight-shaming disguised as progressive ideas about health was in place. People were starting to get wise to the fact that diets don't work, and the diet industry was trying to adapt and stay afloat, as I explain in my first book, *Anti-Diet*. At the same time, writers like Michael

Pollan and Eric Schlosser were opining about America as a "republic of fat" created by fast and processed food (an argument I unpack and critique in *Anti-Diet*), and the more blatant and straightforward diet culture exemplified by companies like WeightWatchers and Jenny Craig was giving way to "it's not a diet, it's a lifestyle." With the rise of rhetoric about the so-called obesity epidemic, dieting began to be framed as an issue of health and wellness—and indeed a matter of life and death—rather than simply as a question of aesthetics.

In the decades since, the increasing entanglement of diet and wellness culture and the pervasive refrain that restrictive eating is the path to wellness have made it much harder to distinguish between harmful trends and what's legitimately beneficial for your well-being.

In order to disentangle those threads, it can be useful to step back and look at the history of wellness as a concept. That could be an entire book on its own, since movements to promote prevention and "natural" healing have existed for centuries. The late 1800s, for example, saw the birth of four major schools of thought that help make up what we now know as alternative (or increasingly "complementary" or "integrative") medicine: naturopathy, homeopathy, osteopathy, and chiropractic. Other modalities that now influence wellness culture, such as Ayurveda, are even older. But the modern incarnation of wellness culture—and its deep entrenchment with diet culture—can be traced back to a series of developments in the 1950s through 1970s. Examining that history will allow us to understand some of the biggest problems with wellness culture today.

### The Birth of Wellness

The term "wellness" first entered the lexicon in the 1650s (as an antonym for "illness"), but the word didn't take on its current meaning until more than 300 years later. That's when medical doctor and public health researcher Halbert Dunn introduced the term "high-level wellness," in a series of lectures and scientific journal articles. Dunn defined wellness in the late 1950s as "an integrated method of functioning which is oriented toward maximizing the potential of which the individual is capable, within the environment where he is functioning."[1] In other words, he saw wellness as an ongoing process of optimizing individual health. For Dunn, high-level wellness was about constantly seeking to improve yourself in the physical, mental, spiritual, and social dimensions, no matter your circumstances. "This definition does not imply that there is an optimum level of wellness, but rather that wellness is a direction in progress toward an ever-higher potential of functioning," he wrote, though the same year he argued that there was such a thing as "peak wellness," a goal that "represents the extreme opposite of death, that is, performance at full potential in accordance with the individual's age and makeup."[2] Dunn also made a distinction between health (the absence of illness) and wellness (an active pursuit of improvement), and defined wellness as involving "the total individual"—mind, body, spirit, and environment.

Despite his notable emphasis on the mental, spiritual, social, and environmental aspects of well-being, and on the importance of human interconnection, Dunn's repeated reference to the individual presages the individualism at the heart of wellness culture. It's a very American ideal, and one that's central to diet culture as well: if an individual fails to meet the standards of beauty and health laid out by the culture, it's their personal responsibility to change their eating and shrink their body in order to fit. And if the diet doesn't work, it's the individual's fault—not the diet's.

But Dunn didn't actually talk much about food and exercise—that would come in later iterations of wellness that built on his work. Instead, he stuck largely to observations about the importance of psychological and emotional factors, which he argued were sorely neglected then—as they are today. In the 1961 book *High-Level Wellness* (a collection of all Dunn's writings and speeches on the topic), he barely mentions food, except to talk about the importance of having enough of it. Far from being a critic of "processed" food, he writes favorably about the role of science in creating an abundant food supply, and he points to the agricultural revolution and food industrialization as having contributed to greater longevity. There's also very little weight stigma in his written work, aside from one small comment in his book ("the most important example of stored energy is fat, of which many of us have a surplus, because we like our food so much"). But even with that remark, his view of fatness seems to be relatively benign—he's not saying that body fat is bad for health, simply that it's a common and notable form of stored energy. The vast majority of his attention seems to be devoted not to food, exercise, or body size—as in wellness culture today—but to the mental and social aspects of well-being. Though Dunn's writing is still a product of its time (with some very 1950s ideas about gender roles within families, for example), many of his ideas about wellness strike me as surprisingly balanced and astute.

The concept of wellness wasn't Dunn's main claim to fame, at least not in his lifetime. He was better known for leading the charge to establish a national health statistics system in the U.S., and he served as chief of the National Office of Vital Statistics (now called the National Center for Health Statistics) from 1935 to 1960. As influential as he was in certain public health circles, his work on wellness didn't reach a wide audience.

Flash forward to 1972, toward the end of Dunn's life. A young medical resident named John Travis walked into a bookstore on the Johns Hopkins University campus in Baltimore and discovered Dunn's book on a clearance table. Intrigued, he bought it, took it home, and started reading. At first, he was not a fan of Dunn's terminology. "I thought the word *wellness* was stupid, and it would never catch on," he told the *New York Times* in 2010.[3] But he liked Dunn's ideas, particularly his promotion of a positive vision of health (rather than simply the avoidance of illness) and his consideration of the whole person. Travis began to implement those concepts in his work and eventually came to accept the word "wellness," too. Around three and a half years after that serendipitous discovery in the bookstore, Travis — by then a fully licensed medical doctor in private practice — opened a facility called the Wellness Resource Center in Mill Valley, California.

At the time, in 1975 (coincidentally the year of Dunn's death), wellness was still such a new concept that Travis often had to spell out the word over the phone. But soon it started to attract national media attention. First, in 1976, a health researcher and fellow Dunn fan named Donald B. Ardell profiled the Wellness Resource Center for *Prevention* magazine. In a sidebar to the piece, the magazine's editor promised that going forward, the magazine would "examine all aspects of wellness promotion." Then, in 1979, wellness hit the mainstream when *60 Minutes* did a segment on it, focusing on Travis and his center. "Wellness," host Dan Rather intones at the top of the segment. "There's a word you don't hear every day."

The segment follows two clients at Travis's center who, having been let down by traditional medical care, apparently found healing through the program and its focus on stress reduction, physical activity, and newer technologies like biofeedback. At this point, Rather asks Travis an important question: Is wellness meant to be "a substitute practice of medicine?" "Absolutely not," Travis replies. "It is an adjunct to, and quite different from, the practice of medicine." Later in the segment, Rather sits in a room full of healthcare professionals who've come to the Wellness Resource Center to learn. A young woman with a brown ponytail says, "Well, I don't like labels, especially with all the latest publicity on cults in the San Francisco area." (Jonestown, Synanon, and the Berkeley Psychic Institute had all been widely covered and called out as cults in 1978 and '79.)[4] "And I think that wellness as a concept doesn't need to have a culture or subculture added to it."[5]

In the twenty-first century, of course, wellness has *become* an entire culture—one that has restrictive eating practices as a central element. Dunn barely spoke about nutrition, and Travis included it only as one part of a multifaceted conception of wellness, one that involved a focus on the mind, stress reduction, communication, and other social factors. Today, however, some alternative and integrative-medicine practitioners seem to focus almost exclusively on diet, and many definitions of "holistic" health are really just about physical interventions like food, exercise, and supplements. Indeed, wellness culture is largely synonymous with diet culture in its approach to food, exercise, and body size. That's not to say that wellness culture entirely ignores other areas of health and healthcare (as we'll discuss in subsequent chapters). But its most visible aspect—and often the first one people encounter—is its teachings about food.

How did that happen? When did wellness culture become so fixated on food?

That shift took place quite early, driven by both the emerging popularity of wellness and the preexisting cultural fixation on physical health. "During the 1970s, ideas about holistic wellness—the notion that individuals should strive for more than the absence of illness, and that body, mind, and to some, spirit, are intertwined—gained wide currency," says Natalia Mehlman Petrzela, the author of *Fit Nation* and a historian at The New School who studies fitness and wellness culture. "Initially, this was expressed primarily in enthusiasm for therapies and practices considered 'alternative' to Western medicine, [but] as these ideas spread, they came to encompass what had been considered the purely physical pursuits of diet and exercise." It was probably inevitable that in a culture that already lionized physical health and didn't have much use for the other dimensions of well-being, discussions of wellness would come to focus on the physical.

The 1970s were also a time when countercultural ideas about food filtered into the mainstream. When Dunn came up with the idea of high-level wellness more than a decade earlier, many people shared his sense that large-scale food production was generally a good thing. But the social upheaval of the late '60s and early '70s started to change that. Young radicals began to question all kinds of American institutions, eventually including the food system. They wanted to make a clean break with the 1950s convenience foods they'd grown up on, rejecting anything packaged or refined, and turning toward alternatives from far outside the white American mainstream like brown rice, granola, yogurt, tofu—all fairly run-of-the-mill today, but totally out-there in the early 1970s, as Jonathan Kauffman explains in *Hippie Food*, his cultural history of that time.[6]

Soon these ideas about food began to catch on with a wider audience. Frances Moore Lappé's book *Diet for a Small Planet* (a political manifesto advocating vegetarianism, with recipes) sold a million copies between 1971 and 1977, Kauffman reports, becoming one of the most influential books of the era. J. I. Rodale, the publisher of *Prevention* and *Organic Gardening and Farming*, had been spreading his unconventional ideas about health—including, most notably, the notion that unprocessed foods were more nutritious than processed ones—to a fairly niche readership since the 1950s, but in the early 1970s the circulation of Rodale's magazines grew significantly and started to reach a younger demographic. People were newly receptive to critiques of the food industry and arguments that "whole" foods were healthier.

That influence is clear in Donald Ardell's 1977 *High Level Wellness: An Alternative to Doctors, Drugs, and Disease*, perhaps the earliest work positioning food as central to wellness. In the book—which became a bestseller and is often credited with launching the wellness movement—Ardell references Dunn's work and credits him for the title. But Ardell leans far more heavily on food than Dunn ever did, making nutrition and physical activity two of his five "dimensions of high-level wellness." In discussing nutrition, Ardell paints foods as good and bad in a way that exemplifies one of the hallmarks of diet culture, calling packaged and processed foods "porno foods" and writing that refined sugar is "worse than no food at all." His description of his own diet and exercise regimen sounds surprisingly similar to the diets of clients I've treated for disordered eating in recent years, particularly those with a type called *orthorexia*, or obsession with "healthy" eating.[7] Indeed, he acknowledges that he's often perceived as a "health nut." Ardell also makes some shockingly fatphobic comments, including advising readers not to listen to higher-weight doctors because of their body size. "By all means discount not just the counsel of such doctors, but also your relationship with them," he writes.[8]

Ardell's book helped embed diet culture in the definition of wellness, and from there, it spread far and wide. By the 1990s, people generally understood "wellness" to mean not only alternative-health modalities like Chinese medicine or meditation, but also food and exercise practices like buying organic vegetables and taking power yoga classes, Petrzela says. Nutrition and physical activity had fully infiltrated the wellness space, which also became a convenient marketing tool for purveyors of diet culture. "The diet and fitness industries were quick to claim the language of 'holistic wellbeing' because it invested the bodily work [they] sold with loftier purpose," she says. A major criticism of those industries had always been that spending on dieting and fitness was superficial, even narcissistic—but making the case that those practices were necessary for overall well-being and thriving was "much higher ground to stand on," she says. Though it was unknown to many people at the time, diet culture also stems in part from racist ideas about white bodies being thinner and therefore better, as sociologist Sabrina Strings explains in her 2019 book *Fearing the Black Body*.[9] But with the rise of wellness culture, dieting and exercise could be reframed not as simply aesthetic or selfish pursuits, but as a matter of attaining your full potential—mentally, emotionally, and spiritually.

In *Anti-Diet* I wrote that wellness culture is the new guise of diet culture, but I've come to understand that there's a symbiotic relationship between the two: from the 1970s onward, wellness culture has incorporated diet culture's tenets as its own, while diet culture uses "wellness" as justification for its existence and a cloak to cover its problematic past. That symbiosis is still thriving today, in ways that have caused tremendous damage to people's relationships with food and their bodies.

### The Perils of the Wellness Diet

Dawn Serra has a calming presence, with kind eyes and an insightful, nonjudgmental demeanor that lend themselves well to her chosen profession as a therapist specializing in body acceptance and trauma. Where other people would say "but," she tends to say "and," a gently drawn-out syllable aimed at complicating simple binaries and acknowledging the complexity of things. Her warm smile and rich laugh make her easy to connect with, but she didn't always feel very connected to herself. She was conditioned to feel bad about her larger body size from a young age, and that infected the way she saw herself. "So much of my story has been 'I'm not worthy,'" she says. "I'm not worthy of love unless XYZ, or I'm not good enough in this body that I'm in."

As she grew up, in the early 1980s through the mid-'90s, one of the things that made her feel unworthy was the increasing rhetoric about the so-called obesity epidemic, which linked higher weight to illness and mortality. So when she discovered wellness culture in her twenties, "It felt like someone had finally told me, 'if you do all of these things you'll never get sick and die,'" she says. She realizes now that she had unconsciously been looking for that holy grail for years. "As someone in a fat body, [for whom] literally the word used to describe my body was *death*, that [sense] of control felt really important."

One of the ways wellness culture entraps us is by promising to stave off death. Sometimes this promise is quite literal, as in the title of the popular wellness-diet book *How Not to Die*.[10] Awareness of our own mortality is terrifying, and at a certain point many of us start looking for some way to evade it. In a world overrun with choices about what to eat and how to move your body (not to mention which skin care products to buy and how to clean your home) — and in an era when such choices can feel freighted not just with responsibility for our own health but also for the fate of the earth itself — wellness culture offers the certainty that if we just follow its rules to the letter, we (and our planet) will be safe. Never mind that those rules are arcane, ever-changing, and wildly inaccessible to most people. Wellness culture claims to be all about "discovering what works for you" by choosing from a perpetually expanding menu of options, the vast majority of which are restrictive in one way or another. Stick to those restrictions and you'll stay alive, it implicitly promises; stray from them and you'll die.

Wellness culture doesn't just guarantee that it will help you fend off illness and death; it also offers the hope that it will enable you to ward off stigma and control how others see you. Pursuing wellness, Serra says, helped her avoid the "bad fatty" stereotype. When people saw her walking around with her green juices, only using organic products, and eschewing plastic, it sent the message that although she was larger-bodied, she was trying her hardest not to be — and in fact was doing more "healthy" behaviors than most thin people. Serra threw herself into research on wellness, learning all she could about amino acids, minerals, pH levels, household chemicals. "I was like a walking encyclopedia," she says. She could feel people's respect and admiration when she spouted her wellness knowledge, and in a sense, it felt like reclaiming the moral high ground. "I felt like I knew something that nobody else knew, and I could judge the people who were often judging me," she says. "Like 'I'm doing more than all of you in thin bodies. So, one, you can't say anything to me because I'm doing all the right things, and two, I feel sorry for you. Look at how you're poisoning your body!' I mean, I was pretty preachy about it," she says.

In wellness culture there's no shortage of sources preaching about food in particular, which is why for many people, the first foray into wellness culture is trying to change what they eat in order to feel better — an understandable goal, given how much that idea is pushed on us by media and social media, Western and alternative-medicine practitioners alike. The problem is that often it's not a particularly safe or effective goal. Cutting out food groups, restricting your eating to certain times of day, or otherwise overhauling your menu is a big deal for most people — a major life change that can divide you from friends, family, and culture and interfere with your ability to take pleasure or find spontaneity in food.

Changing what you eat is especially risky if you already have a fraught relationship with food, which I would say most people in Western culture do. Women and transgender people are disproportionately affected. One survey found that some 75 percent of women between the ages of 25 and 45 have some form of disordered eating, including 10 percent who met the clinical criteria for full-blown eating disorders, though far fewer are actually diagnosed.[11] The percentage may be even higher in transgender populations, according to several studies.[12] Cisgender men, too, are struggling with food issues in increasing numbers. A 2019 study found that nearly a quarter of young men aged 18–24 have signs of disordered eating—specifically "muscularity-oriented disordered eating behaviors," which include eating more or differently to try to bulk up.[13] And the overall prevalence of eating disorders among men and women in the U.S., Europe, and Asia more than doubled between 2000 and 2018.[14]

When people are starting from a place of anxiety about food, restricting and radically altering their intake in the name of wellness can lead to more intensely disordered eating. That can be true even for people who had never dieted before.

Take a reader of mine named Jaime, who shared that her doctor recommended an elimination diet to address her health concerns, which included acne, IBS, headaches, and depression. Prior to that diet, never in her 27 years of life had she been on a diet to lose weight, and she didn't feel much stress or anxiety around eating. But all of that changed when she went on the elimination diet. "While the goal of the diet at the outset was not to lose weight, by the end it became my sole focus," Jaime wrote to me in 2020. The diet was so restrictive that it made it impossible to eat enough, so she lost a lot of weight very quickly—and got a surprising onslaught of compliments from friends, family, and strangers alike, sending the message that her body was only acceptable and desirable at this new lower weight. "Now—although I have reintroduced almost all food groups, and I'm trying to return to normalcy—I am still restricting calories and have found myself obsessed with my body and trying to maintain its new weight," she wrote. Her once peaceful relationship with food and her body morphed into extreme anxiety around food and weight gain. What's more, the diet didn't even work for its stated purpose, as is the case for many people who embark on wellness-culture diets (as we'll discuss in Chapter 5). "My digestive system got progressively worse over the course of the elimination diet, with severe simultaneous diarrhea, constipation, and constant bloating," she wrote.

Serra found herself in a similar predicament when she began eliminating foods. "The whole thing starts with cutting out processed foods, and then it goes to trying to make everything fruits and veggies, and then it goes to juice," she says. "And then for a while I was as far into raw as I could go." She says by that point, she was regularly "cheating" by eating larger portions than recommended, simply because she felt so hungry all the time—which is the body's natural response to not getting enough food, and an all-too-common experience among dieters. "But I thought it was a 'me' thing, of course," she says. Wellness culture, like diet culture, makes failure out to be the individual's fault.

That's a problem not just because it's misleading, but also because it keeps people locked in a disordered cycle with food. When you're following food rules, whether you're cognizant of it or not, they often start to take over your life. That happened for Serra, and she still feels the effects even though she's been firmly committed to recovery for years. To this day, when she eats foods that she knows aren't wellness culture–approved, "there are some loud voices inside me saying 'if you take one bite of that, you're going to die,'" she says. And "okay, you took a bite—don't take that second bite, or you're going to die." Although she'd been dieting for decades by the time she discovered wellness culture, she'd never had that kind of anxiety about particular foods. "I mean, I had anxiety just because I was moving through the world in a bigger body, but getting involved with these wellness spaces really took it to a particularly nasty level," she says. In many ways, wellness culture caused her more harm than traditional diet culture. And that damage is more enduring as well. "It makes me really angry knowing I'm probably going to continue to have that be a part of my experience for a long time," she says.

Wellness culture doesn't advertise those risks, but they're very real. "I think it's a perspective a lot of people have that when you do dietary changes in particular, you think, 'what's the harm? It's just food,'" Maxine Ali says. But the reality is that changing your diet in the restrictive ways that wellness culture demands can have a profound impact on your physical and mental health. And it's something that far too few people are talking about. "I very much just wish that there had been someone aware of this to say, 'is this the best idea?'" Ali says. It's a question we'd all do well to ask ourselves and our loved ones when it comes to dieting, or really anything wellness related. Wellness practices often seem less risky to people because they're not explicitly called diets, but it's important to know that they can do just as much damage as traditional diets, if not more.

### Juicing and Cleansing

One of Serra's big investments in wellness culture was buying an expensive "masticating" juicer that was supposed to somehow leave the nutrients more intact than the lower-end centrifugal juicer she had, which apparently "killed" the nutrients by heating them. That's an understandable assumption—nutrients like vitamin C and other antioxidants are indeed somewhat sensitive to heat from cooking—but it turns out it's not necessarily true when it comes to different juicing methods. Several studies have found that there's no significant difference in the nutrient content of juice produced by centrifugal juicers and masticating juicers (better known today as cold-press juicers).[15] In fact, one study with grape juice found that juicing methods that heated the juice ended up producing a *greater* amount of antioxidants and other beneficial compounds than cold-pressing.[16] That's not even to mention the fact that juicing doesn't have any special benefits that you wouldn't get just by eating fruits and vegetables, cooked or raw—and many fruits and vegetables contain nutrients that are *only* unlocked through cooking. What's more, those beautiful bottles of cold-pressed juices that you see in wellness stores and on Instagram are more likely to harbor bacteria that cause foodborne illness than are the pasteurized juices found in refrigerated sections of supermarkets.

Yet the pressure to juice — or "juice-cleanse" — and to have all the right equipment for it continues, demonstrating some of the classism inherent in wellness culture. It's a huge expense to buy fancy, wellness-y juices at upwards of $10 a bottle, and domestic cold-press juicers run from hundreds of dollars to several thousand — and then you need to factor in the ongoing price of raw materials. "I didn't do juice cleanses regularly because I couldn't really afford to," Ali says, "but when I had that kind of money to put away, I did." It's much more expensive to produce a serving of juice than it is to just cook up some veggies: often pounds of produce need to go into a juicer for one glass (which probably won't even make a satisfying breakfast on its own, let alone a lunch or dinner), whereas those same ingredients likely could stretch across several meals otherwise. Keeping vegetables relatively intact rather than pressing them down into juice retains the fiber, too (though fiber isn't the nutritional panacea it's often made out to be in diet and wellness culture). "Greens powders," a more recent addition to the wellness market, are cheaper per serving than standard green juice but still relatively expensive for something that can't serve as a meal on its own.

Green juice first exploded on the wellness scene in the early 2010s, but by the following decade it was all about specific *kinds* of green juice. There was a phase during which it was seen as superior if you could drink (and tolerate) bitter green juices rather than those sweetened with apple, orange, or other sweet fruits. It wasn't just about added sugar anymore; now even the sugar in fruit was considered bad. As I write this, the trend is celery juice, promoted by a Gwyneth Paltrow–endorsed wellness personality who calls himself the Medical Medium. Born Anthony

William Coviello, the Medical Medium has no medical or scientific training or credentials. He claims that since he was four
years old he's been channeling a spirit (which he calls "the Spirit
of Compassion," or simply "the Spirit") that gives health diagnoses and wellness advice that modern science supposedly isn't
advanced enough to corroborate. The Spirit is communicated
to him by a voice that ostensibly told him in the late 1970s (when
cold-pressed juice was very much not a trend) to start recommending celery juice to family and friends with various ailments. Now, some five decades later, he's pushing it as a cure-all
for everything from acne to addiction, chronic pain to cancer,
without any evidence to support these wild claims.

If William were a medical professional he'd be in danger of
losing his license, but ironically he's protected by the fact that
he has no credentials. He's called celery juice a "miracle tonic,"[17]
harking back to the old-timey snake-oil salesmen that we'll discuss in Chapter 7. And he has an audience of millions—a disturbingly large reach for someone making such implausible
claims—thanks in considerable part to the support of Paltrow
and a number of other high-profile celebrities who have no wellness credentials to speak of, plus the amplification of social
media algorithms that privilege novelty and controversy above
nuance and solid evidence. Indeed, the fact that William's ideas
are so out-there is likely a large part of the reason they succeed
online, as we'll discuss in Chapter 4.

I find William's rhetoric particularly troubling because his
laundry list of illnesses that celery juice supposedly cures includes
nearly all of the ones I have, including autoimmune diseases, IBS,
and allergies—and there was a point in my life when I was so
desperate for help and healing that I probably would have drunk
the juice of one or two entire bunches of celery every day (his
recommended dose) on an uncredentialed influencer's orders.
Millions of people are in that same place right now, vulnerable
and searching for answers. Unfortunately, at best they're likely

just wasting time and money, and at worst they're doing themselves real harm.

There are unintended consequences to mega-dosing celery juice, as there are with consuming such large amounts of pretty much anything, including creating some of the very symptoms William claims the juice can cure. For one thing, it can worsen gastrointestinal issues: Like some other trendy juices, celery juice can have a diuretic effect for people with sensitive GI tracts, which are one of the key groups to whom William pitches it. To be clear, the diarrhea you will likely get from consuming two cups of celery juice before breakfast isn't "toxins leaving your body"—it's just dehydrating and painful. Drinking large amounts of celery juice can also potentially trigger an allergy to the vegetable, and reactions to celery are relatively common in some areas: Within the European Union, for example, celery is one of the 14 foods that must be declared as allergens on food labels.[18] Moreover, drinking large amounts of celery juice can also make you more sensitive to ultraviolet A light, thanks to compounds in celery called psoralens. Although exposure to UVA rays in controlled settings may help improve the symptoms of skin conditions like psoriasis and eczema, it can also damage the skin and increase the risk of skin cancer.[19]

Juice cleanses are still a big trend—and big business. But as more attention has been paid to the restrictive nature of these cleanses in recent years, a new type of cleanse has come on the scene: the "whole-food cleanse," of the kind often sold by fancy home meal-delivery services. These cleanses are still expensive and restrictive, still very much a part of wellness-diet culture, but less *obviously* diet-y than strictly juice-based cleanses—which helps them appeal to a growing number of people who want something seemingly a little more flexible, more intuitive, than a traditional cleanse or detox. They're diets for people who want to eat solid foods instead of just drink liquids, but diets nonetheless.

In recent years, a new version of diets disguised as wellness plans has emerged: "intuitive fasting." Pushed by another of Gwyneth Paltrow's associates, intuitive fasting is a version of intermittent fasting that claims to be less restrictive and seems to want to appeal more to the crunchy center of the wellness world than to the hard, gym-and-tech-bro edges. Though it co-opts the language of intuitive eating, intuitive fasting is totally out of alignment with true intuitive eating, which is an anti-diet approach whose first principle is to reject the diet mentality. Of course people are free to sell diets—and go on diets—as much as they want, but it's important to call them what they really are. There's nothing intuitive about a diet that tells you when, what, and how much (or how often) you're allowed to eat. What's more, fasting is actually an eating-disorder behavior. One of the first few uses of the phrase "intermittent fasting" in scientific research on humans is in a 1996 case study of behaviors in a patient with an eating disorder.[20] Use of the term "intuitive fasting" is just another example of wellness culture presenting disordered eating behaviors as harmless pathways to better health, with potentially devastating consequences for people's relationships with food and their bodies.

In fact, that was the case for Paltrow's own former chief content officer at *goop*, Elise Loehnen. In a 2022 Instagram post, she shared that doing repeated cleanses during her *goop* years "distorted" her relationship with her body, and that for her cleansing became "synonymous with dieting and restriction."[21] When she left the company in 2020, it helped her see that "wellness culture can be toxic," and she vowed never to do a cleanse again. Yet in the post where she revealed all of this, she was already promoting another cleanse—a "five-day reset of broths, smoothies, and lattes"—and said she'd likely follow it up with a fast.

This about-face isn't all that surprising, because once you've come under wellness culture's intense pressure to cleanse and restrict your eating, it can be hard to find true balance again. In an ideology that paints foods as good and bad and frames cutting out food groups as the path to good health, there's not a lot of room for a relaxed, peaceful relationship with food.

### Animal Wellness

The unintended consequences of wellness culture don't just affect us humans; increasingly they also seem to be impacting the other animals in our midst. In recent years, veterinarians have noted a rise in the incidence of a serious heart condition called dilated cardiomyopathy (DCM) in dogs fed what the ASPCA calls "boutique, exotic, grain-free" food. As of this writing, the U.S. Food and Drug Administration (FDA) is still investigating the link, but it notes that of the products fed to animals who suffered from DCM, "more than 90 percent...were 'grain-free,' and 93 percent...had peas and/or lentils."[22] A sea of wellness terms—"natural," "nature," "holistic," "wild"—can be found in the marketing copy and lists of ingredients for the brands whose products' names crop up in the reports being studied by the FDA.

For many pets, there really doesn't seem to be a need for grain-free food in the first place. As the World Small Animal Veterinary Association notes, "dogs and cats can digest cereal grains if they are properly cooked and as long as the overall diet is complete and balanced, and there is no evidence to show they are harmful for our pets."[23] So why did the trend start? Kathryn Michel, a professor of animal nutrition at the University of Pennsylvania School of Veterinary Medicine, told *NBC News* that trends in pet foods tend to follow those seen in human food. "So while I don't know 100 percent where the grain-free idea started from, it started cropping up when people started embracing low-carb diets and gluten-free foods," she said.[24]

The incursion of wellness culture into animals' lives isn't just limited to pets. El Poché, a former member of my admin team who also volunteers at a wildlife rehabilitation center, remembers seeing a squirrel that was brought into the center after the person who found it gave it a homeopathic treatment they'd found on the Internet. Poché says that the person incorrectly diagnosed the squirrel with parasites and then followed the online advice to syringe-feed the animal a mixture of honey and water to supposedly purge the bugs. "Needless to say, all of this was ill-advised, and ultimately the squirrel had to be humanely euthanized," they told me in an email. "It's a familiar occurrence these days, and is a cause of great frustration to wildlife rehab organizations."

Erin Lemley, a wildlife veterinary technician on staff at the program where Poché volunteers, notes that she's also seen an increase in "alternative therapies" being discussed at professional events in the field, such as a recent conference presentation that advocated using essential oils on wildlife patients—who are typically in rehab for serious conditions such as neurological trauma, broken bones, or lead toxicity. In the slide deck from that presentation, under "Why Essential Oils?" the first bullet point is "Raise Frequency of Animal" (more on "frequencies" and "vibrations" in Chapter 3). It goes on to recommend feeding animals the oils with toothpicks or placing oils directly in the mouth or on food, "spray-bottle misting" for reptiles and birds, and using the "petting method" (which ostensibly means putting oil on your hand and petting the animal) for animals with dense fur.

The presenter wasn't a veterinarian or even a registered aromatherapist, but a distributor for Young Living—a multilevel-marketing company that sells essential oils.

### Getting Torched

Right alongside the restrictive and dangerous food practices at the center of wellness culture are problematic exercise regimens. Although some forms of physical activity skew crunchy, like certain yoga classes, often there's a much harsher energy to the fitness world. Even wellness websites with feminine, millennial-pink aesthetics have articles in their fitness sections about "booty burning," "torching those abs," and "lighting your glutes and legs on fire." And often what all of that really means, even if it's never overtly stated, is getting thinner.

"I joined a gym, I think, for the reason a lot of people do: I just wanted to lose weight," says Chrissy King, author of *The Body Liberation Project*. Now a fitness and strength coach who's firmly against diet culture, King first started working out simply because she thought it would make her thin. "I remember I hired a trainer and I told her, 'make me skinny.' That was my sole purpose for getting into fitness."

In response, the trainer gave her a low-calorie diet that provided less than half of what her body's actual energy needs probably were. Granted, King hadn't told her that she was doing cardio workouts in addition to their strength-training sessions, and in any case the trainer only wanted her to stay on the diet for a month. But King now recognizes that no matter what, it was harmful for the trainer to advise anyone to eat so little. "I saw quick results, so of course I just kept doing it," she says. She became so controlling with food that a few times, when she ate a little more than she thought she should, she felt so guilty that she engaged in bulimic behaviors. Though she was never diagnosed with an eating disorder, she can see now how harmful that diet was to her well-being, and how disordered her relationship with food became. "I think the fitness industry is really, really good at preying on people's insecurities, and at the base of all insecurities around fitness is weight," she says.

While the bulimic behaviors did serve as something of a wake-up call that she needed to stop being so obsessive about food and her body, she couldn't let go of dieting altogether. She just switched to other diets that were slightly less restrictive, and she remained fixated on food and her body, continuing to struggle with disordered eating for several more years. "People were constantly complimenting me on my body everywhere I went, but I was probably the most self-conscious about my body that I'd ever been," she says. "I look back at those pictures now and I can see how thin I was, but at the time I would look in the mirror and pick my body apart."

King was lucky in that she never developed any serious health issues, either during her disordered-eating phase or before or since. Many people do develop significant health problems when they're overexercising and/or undereating, but for King, no matter what size she's been or how much she's moved her body (or not), she's always been in good physical health. But because of wellness-culture rhetoric, when she was working out compulsively she started to believe that was the *reason* she wasn't ill—that exercise alone was responsible for keeping her well. "My mindset around health was definitely based on what you look like and not, you know, acknowledging the fact that I had a horrible issue with food, I had a horrible issue with my body image, I had a horrible issue with exercise," she says. "I was like, 'I've achieved health and I look the part. And if everybody else had the same kind of discipline as me, they also would have similar outcomes to me.'"

This line of thinking exemplifies the wellness-culture myth that if you "look well," it must be because you are. But often, as King can attest, nothing could be further from the truth. People who appear physically "healthy" may in fact be grappling with serious mental-health problems such as disordered eating and body obsession, as King was, not to mention depression, anxiety, or other issues. In fact, looking "well" according to wellness culture can sometimes be one of the only external signs that you're seriously struggling. By no means am I encouraging people to go around judging each other by their looks, but in my experience, for most people the particular look that wellness culture lionizes can only be attained through compulsive exercise and restrictive eating. What's held up as the picture of health in wellness culture is often actually the hallmark of a deeply disordered relationship with food and movement.

It's also exclusionary: it doesn't include people with disabilities, larger-bodied people, and most people who are middle-aged or older; it rarely includes people of color or other marginalized groups. This is evident in the structure and makeup of fitness spaces. Not only are gyms often lacking in accessibility for people with disabilities, but many are also inaccessible to transgender people because they lack gender-neutral changing rooms and bathrooms. They're also often financially inaccessible: Before the pandemic, the average monthly gym membership cost fifty-eight dollars, and it was common to see boutique fitness classes in the jaw-dropping range of thirty to forty-five dollars for a single class in major cities.[25] The lack of ethnic diversity in fitness spaces may be partly related to those costs, but it's also undoubtedly influenced by a lack of representation. "When you look at fitness overall, as far as I can see, it's always been marketed to thin, cis, able-bodied people, white people," says King, who is Black. Although today there are some notable examples of non-white, non-able-bodied fitness instructors with large national presences, the average local gym is still likely to advertise with images of muscular white guys. "And when we look at the cover of fitness magazines, when we look at major fitness outlets and the platforms that are known to be leaders in the fitness industry, it's overwhelmingly white, overwhelmingly male. We just don't see representation of people of different backgrounds," King says.

What's more, there have been many examples of overt racism and other forms of discrimination in the fitness industry. In June of 2020, the founder and former CEO of CrossFit, Greg Glassman, posted a tweet that managed to mock both the COVID-19 pandemic and the murder of George Floyd, and he then doubled down on this rhetoric in a belligerent Zoom call with CrossFit gym owners about race and racism. "We're not mourning for George Floyd, I don't think me or any of my staff are," he said on that call, according to a recording leaked to the *New York Times*.[26] "Can you tell me why I should mourn for him?" he said. "Other than it's the 'white' thing to do. I get that pressure, but give me another reason." Glassman resigned as Cross-Fit CEO amid public outcry, and a few weeks later he sold the company to a new owner. Meanwhile, *Business Insider* reported in November of 2020 that numerous SoulCycle instructors have made racist remarks to class participants, in addition to using homophobic language, making unwanted sexual advances, and fat-shaming employees.[27]

Today, King does significantly less physical activity (and weighs significantly more) than she did in her compulsive-exercise days, and her physical health hasn't changed. The only thing that has is her mental health and her relationship with food, movement, and her body, which have all improved markedly. "I'm just so much more grounded and actually paying attention to what my body feels like doing and what it needs," she says. She's moved away from the performative fitness that's often shown on social media—how many reps you did, how long you ran, before-and-after photos. "My focus now is on how I'm nourishing my body through exercise or movement, what feels good for me, and what ways are actually adding joy to my life."

That positive relationship with physical activity is available to people of every size. Despite some scientific debate, numerous studies over the past twenty-plus years have shown that it's very much possible to be "fat and fit." For example, a 2017 study of more than five thousand people[28] and a 2014 meta-analysis of ten studies with nearly ninety-three thousand participants[29] found no increased risk of cardiovascular disease or death for physically active higher-weight people. Additionally, a 2021 review of the evidence found that most cardiometabolic risk factors associated with high body mass index (BMI) can be improved with physical activity independent of weight loss, and that increases in cardiore-spiratory fitness or physical activity are consistently associated with *greater* reductions in mortality risk than is intentional weight loss.[30] In wellness culture, "fit" people are pretty much always portrayed as thin—but they don't have to be.


### Biohacking and Tech-Bro Dieting

As a journalist and dietitian who specializes in disordered eat-ing, I make a habit of not going into detail about any diet, because those minutiae can provide a how-to manual for people with eating disorders. So I won't describe exactly what Jack Dorsey eats in a week—but I will say that the Twitter founder seems to consume a disturbingly small amount of food. As he revealed in a 2019 interview, he practices a highly restrictive ver-sion of intermittent fasting that involves eating next to nothing on weekdays, and at one point he was eating even less on week-ends. He said "time slows down" on these extended fasts, which it tends to do when you're starving.[31] Even on weekdays, his intake is probably only about a third of what he needs to support his basic energy needs and his high level of physical activity.

Dorsey is a grown adult who's free to do whatever he wants with his body. But it's important to call this behavior what it is: disordered eating. As I mentioned above, an early appear-ance of the phrase "intermittent fasting" in the scientific litera-ture was in reference to the behaviors of a patient with an eating disorder—a female aviation student, as it happened. If Dorsey were a woman, his behaviors likely would have raised more alarm bells—but because he's a tech bro, his disordered eating gets recast as a powerful productivity hack. In the words of *Washing-ton Post* columnist Monica Hesse, "it's both remarkable and depressing to watch Jack Dorsey blithely describe a diet that would put any woman—or any non-wealthy man—into the penalty box of public opinion."[32] In the early pages of eating-disorder memoirs, there's often a description of the heightened sense of energy and focus—euphoria, even—that comes in the early days of starvation, before all the harmful consequences like passing out, breaking bones, becoming more susceptible to infections, and losing relationships. That's not to mention the increased risk of heart failure from the lack of adequate nourishment, particularly essential minerals like sodium, magnesium, and potassium. The increased productivity that might temporarily accompany fasting isn't worth the long-term consequences.

Yet a disturbing number of Silicon Valley denizens have followed Dorsey into this hellish lifestyle. "Jack Dorsey Is Gwyneth Paltrow for Silicon Valley," a 2019 *New York Times* headline proclaimed, citing his ability to instantly create waiting lists for any wellness product or practice he endorses. "The lithe, 42-year-old tech founder has become a one-man Goop." The former CEO of Evernote told *The Guardian* that getting into fasting was "definitely one of the top two or three most important things I've done in my life."[33] He also shared that he was part of a private WhatsApp group filled with Bay Area CEOs and investors called Fast Club, dedicated to periodic food abstention. Since 2020, Silicon Valley fasters have upped the ante with an even more restrictive diet known as dopamine fasting, which involves eschewing not just food but also any form of mental stimulation, including conversation, music, and even eye contact.

Proponents insist that this type of self-imposed food deprivation is not dieting or disordered eating, but "biohacking"—a wellness trend that targets mostly men with promises of leveled-up productivity and physical performance. Dave Asprey, creator of the "bulletproof" trend of putting butter in your morning coffee, is largely responsible for popularizing biohacking, which he defines as "the process of using science, biology, and self-experimentation to take control of and upgrade your body, mind, and life."[34] While the crunchy heart of wellness culture talks of whole foods and cleanses and *vibrations*, biohacking positions itself as much more scientific. "Biohacking is the art and science of changing the environment around you and inside you so you have more control over your own biology," says Asprey.

The term "biohacking" actually dates back to 1988, when a *Washington Post* article discussed the possibility that literal computer hackers would get into the biotech game, engineering new organisms and sequencing genomes in their basements.[35] Now, thirty-five years later, biohacking is a major wellness trend that has (perhaps unsurprisingly) turned out to be much more of a selfish pursuit than the *Post* predicted. Biohacking adherents seek to "optimize" and constantly improve their own performance through an endless array of interventions: fasting and other esoteric eating and exercise practices, using untested supplements to supposedly "unlock the brain's full potential," obsessively tracking vital signs like body composition (of which body fat is a subcategory) and blood sugar (in the absence of diabetes). Asprey, in his widely publicized quest to live to 180 years old, gets stem-cell infusions, downs more than 150 supplements per day, and tries bizarre treatments to ostensibly ward off aging in various body parts—like getting his penis shot with sound waves. He had that one filmed (from the waist up), and he's wearing a black shirt that says *Upgraded* as he explains how the treatment supposedly works: "It gives you, well, the penis of a very young man as you age. And that's my goal, is to age but not actually age." In an even more extreme biohacking subculture known as grinder, adherents actually implant things into their bodies, like microchips and LEDs, in an effort to increase their capabilities—albeit in very minor ways for now, like eliminating the need for a key fob or flashlight. Grinders hope that once the technology gets good enough, these kinds of hacks can help overcome the fallibilities of the human body and, eventually, enable them to live forever.

As we've discussed, wellness culture in general trades on the often implicit promise of extending life and warding off death. But biohacking makes that pledge explicit, arguing that if you forgo the pleasure of everyday comforts like eating regularly and *not* getting your nether regions shot with weird devices, you'll be rewarded with years of added life and youth. The question is, at what cost? To me, spending hours every day on the hustle of trying to hack your body doesn't seem like the most fulfilling use of your limited time on earth, even if that time is slightly longer as a result of the biohacking techniques you try—and that's a big if.

Indeed, there's no concrete evidence that practices like intermittent fasting have any long-term benefit. Though there have been some small studies linking intermittent fasting to positive effects—and a number of other studies that are highly speculative or that only conducted their research on animals—the results have been mixed and are far too early-stage to justify the hype around the diet. Two randomized controlled trials from 2020 and 2022 found that there was no significant difference in weight loss or cardiometabolic risk factors between intermittent fasting and other diets at either the 12-week or the 12-month mark.[36] The 2022 study, which followed participants for a year and used a standard calorie-restricted diet for the control group, found that on both types of diet people initially lost weight but that it came back over time, and that many of the changes in body composition and metabolic risk factors reverted toward the baseline on both diets as well. Both studies found that people tended to lose muscle mass from intermittent fasting, with the 2020 study finding that fasters lost significantly more muscle than the control group (who were not told to restrict their calorie intake). UCSF cardiologist Ethan Weiss, an author of that study who himself had done intermittent fasting for seven years, said that he was shocked by the findings. "I went into this hoping to demonstrate that this thing I've been doing for years works," Weiss told CNBC.[37] "But as soon as I saw the data, I stopped."

What's more, even if there were benefits to intermittent fasting or other extremely low-calorie diets, it's incredibly difficult for many (I'd argue most) people to stay on those diets long-term without damaging their relationship with food and their mental, emotional, and social well-being. And if a way of eating detracts from those aspects of your life, can it really be called wellness?

While many wellness proponents probably will never try intermittent fasting (let alone implanting microchips into their bodies), one aspect of biohacking that's made its way into mainstream wellness culture is the obsessive tracking and testing of various aspects of health. Fitness trackers have become ever more sophisticated, so that now you can track your blood-oxygen levels and even perform relatively complex tests from anywhere—an Apple Watch commercial shows a man in a boat, floating in a tiny patch of water in the middle of a frozen lake, taking an electrocardiogram. Other wearable devices track sleep, stress levels, and menstrual cycles, in addition to tracking steps.

Some people are even tracking their bowel movements in the name of wellness. "Not only does stool tell you about the health of your diet, but it shows you how your body's digestive system is handling the foods you eat," Dr. Anish Sheth, a Princeton-based gastroenterologist and coauthor of *What's Your Poo Telling You?*, told *Time*.[38] But there are many reasons your poop could look weird. It's not just what you eat and whether or not your body is "handling" it; stress, changes in routine, and disordered eating can also affect your bowel movements, but those things rarely get mentioned in the poop-tracking world. Instead, people are encouraged to hyper-focus on what they're eating and look for possible "intolerances," which can lead to a restrictive and obsessive relationship with food.

The same is true for at-home microbiome and food-intolerance testing kits, which generally aren't based on sound science. Take Everlywell, a home-testing company that makes a "food sensitivity" test that supposedly checks for intolerances to dozens of common food items. In reality, its results likely signal the opposite—that in fact you tolerate those foods perfectly well. That's because it tests for immunoglobulin G (IgG) antibodies, which have specifically been linked to the development of food *tolerance* or desensitization.[39] If your blood contains IgG antibodies to a wide variety of foods, it doesn't mean you have to cut them all out—it simply means you've recently been exposed to those foods. In fact, the very foods you eat most regularly are the ones that tend to show up in IgG tests. I've had numerous clients and audience members tell me, despairingly, that they're "intolerant" to pretty much all the foods they were consuming every day, not realizing that they'd been misled by spurious testing. In wellness culture, the fallibility of IgG tests (and similar problematic tests) isn't common knowledge, and their results are often taken as gospel.

Some home testing kits use different technology, claiming to use your DNA to tell whether you have a food sensitivity. But the genetics of food allergy and intolerance are still very early-stage and correlational, and as the golden rule in statistics goes, correlation is not causation. Just because a gene is linked to a food allergy or intolerance doesn't mean that gene *causes* food sensitivity—or that the gene is even "switched on" for a particular person. So genetic tests generally aren't of much value in diagnosing food sensitivities, as much as diet and wellness culture might condition us to believe otherwise.

In general, "food sensitivity" tests probably aren't going to give you any useful results and may well cause harm by telling you to unnecessarily restrict foods—which is particularly problematic for anyone who already has a fraught relationship with food.

The same is true of "gut-health" tests that purport to tell you the state of your intestinal microbiome and which direct you to diets or supplements to heal it. Granted, laboratory testing for gastrointestinal pathogens can have some value, such as in cases of infection with germs or parasites that are well studied and well known to cause problems. But the science on the gut microbiome as a whole is still in its infancy, and tests that purport to measure it are not approved by the FDA. They test for many microbes that just aren't well understood and shouldn't be used to make diet or supplement recommendations. Even more concerning, they may be riddled with inaccuracies, making them unhelpful for diagnosing anything. For example, in a 2020 study of one such test—the GI-MAP, which is often ordered by functional-medicine doctors—researchers collected human feces that didn't contain any of the bacteria or parasites that the GI-MAP tests for, and used seven samples of that "clean" feces as controls.[40] They then divided the rest of the microbe-free feces into 16 samples and "spiked" each one with one of the germs that the test looks for. The GI-MAP test missed 20 percent of the spiked samples, and it produced false positives for a whopping 74 percent of the samples—meaning it claimed to detect specific microbes where they weren't present at all.

Leaving aside the fact that so many of these tests don't actually work, wellness culture posits that by knowing exactly what's going on in your body, you can "optimize" both physical and mental function, thereby increasing productivity. The fasting part is definitely about thinness for some biohackers—Asprey and others have spoken with pride about losing large amounts of weight—but it's also a nod to the notion that not eating means getting more done. Rob Rhinehart, the founder of Soylent, developed the meal-replacement beverage when he was a twenty-four-year-old programmer living in Silicon Valley because he thought eating was a waste of time. "Not having to worry about food is fantastic," he said in a 2013 interview about subsisting almost entirely on Soylent, which at the time was just a concoction he was making in his kitchen and sharing about on his blog.[41] "I save hours a day and hundreds of dollars a month. I feel liberated from a crushing amount of repetitive drudgery." The time he spent cooking and ordering and chewing food could now be re-allocated to programming—and eventually to his startup, because venture-capital money started flooding in once tech types got wind of this new drink-a-chalky-concoction-instead-of-eating productivity hack. As commenters pointed out soon after the product launched, Soylent is basically just SlimFast with millennial tech-bro branding, and a cheeky name that references a classic sci-fi novel* (not the film adaptation where Soylent was made out of people, Rhinehart is quick to point out). But that branding made all the difference, and young men who wouldn't be caught dead with a SlimFast in their hand came flocking to Soylent.

In the years since, Soylent as a company has grown up a lot. It now has a noble mission that one can hardly imagine coming from a typical diet-shake company: "to make complete, sustainable nutrition accessible, appealing, and affordable to all." It gives money to food banks and homeless shelters and has partnered with World Food Program USA to help fight global malnutrition. Although it can be hard to know for sure with "mission-driven" startups, it seems like Soylent is genuinely helping people with food insecurity.

And yet the reason Soylent exists in the first place—and that biohacking as a whole exists, for that matter—indicates that something is very wrong in the corner of the world where it originated. When people have enough money to afford food but choose not to eat—or feel pressured into that choice by corporate culture—in order to spend more time working, it's a sign that the system is broken. Late-stage capitalism, and the companies that fuel it, are eroding our humanity—our ability to bond and connect over food, to take pleasure in eating, to get out of our heads and into our bodies. They're taking away a truly special ritual shared by human societies the world over. They're turning us into machines and calling it wellness.

---

* *Soylent Green*, by Harry Harrison, no relation (though that is, coincidentally, the name of my cat).

# CHAPTER 2

# Clean and Natural

Dawn Serra, the therapist and former wellness devotee we met in the last chapter, had a relationship with wellness culture that started with food but quickly branched out from there. The creeping sense that everything she ate was full of noxious chemicals led her to start questioning what was in the other everyday items she used, and soon she was only buying organic cleaning products for her home. Then she began to obsess about even more esoteric things. "I started getting really into homesteading and looking at ways that I could, like, make my own towels and make my own dishwasher tablets, because all of those things are filled with these horrible parabens," she says. Products she once took for granted, that made it possible to get through daily chores relatively quickly, were now stumbling blocks to the life of wellness she sought.

Of course there's nothing wrong with seeking out eco-friendly products or making your own (if you have the time and resources to do that, because it often takes a fair amount of both). I've been known to do the occasional DIY household-product project, and I buy as many eco-friendly cleaners as my budget will allow. In fact, my first full-time job was as an editor at a "green" lifestyle magazine.

But just as with food, perfectionism with other aspects of wellness culture can start to interfere with your life — and damage your mental health.

"It really got deep in me that because it was 'morally good' to live life this way, to slip at all was to question your fundamental goodness," Serra says. If she wasn't able to get to Whole Foods to buy her expensive paraben-free, vegan, cruelty-free hand soap and she popped into Target and just grabbed whatever hand soap she could find, she fretted that she was poisoning herself every time she washed her hands. When she ran out of homemade laundry detergent and used a store-bought variety, she worried that her clothes were now covered in "cancer-causing chemicals."

The idea that what you put on your skin or bring into your home will make or break your health has become as much a hallmark of wellness culture as the idea that every bite of food you eat will hurt or heal you. It's often framed as being an easy switch—just avoid these "toxic" foods/products and use these "safe" ones instead—but the implications of not being able to follow wellness culture's every rule are stark. "If you're being given the secrets to living forever and never getting sick, that means to break from that is to be killing yourself," Serra says.

For many people, wellness culture's views on food are a gateway into a belief system where every product is a potential threat, every lifestyle choice a matter of life and death. What starts as "clean eating"—a term that's somewhat fallen out of vogue when it comes to food, because it's justifiably been criticized for its moralistic overtones—often leads into "clean beauty" and "clean lifestyle" (terms that, thus far, still seem to be accepted in the wellness world). It can slide further into a belief that herbal and dietary supplements are safer than medications because they're more "natural," despite the fact that the supplement industry is largely unregulated and supplements may be contaminated with drugs and other substances. This elevation of all things "natural" at the heart of wellness culture can lead people to eschew lifesaving medications and rely instead on untested and harmful supplements and wellness practices.

## Inside and Out

One of the most egregious of wellness culture's damaging assumptions is that if you're really making all the "right" choices, it will show on the outside, in the form of adherence to conventional beauty standards. If you deviate from those standards at all—by, say, having acne, dry skin, brittle hair, or any of the other myriad human characteristics that wellness culture (and Western culture in general) considers "flaws"—then that means you're not truly *well* on the inside. It means you must be doing something wrong, must not be doing wellness well enough—and must need to buy more of the myriad products that the wellness industry is right there to sell you when you have this realization.

Indeed, "beauty starts within" is the underlying philosophy of countless ads for wellness-y products and pills. Makeup magnate Bobbi Brown wrote a wellness book called *Beauty from the Inside Out*, launched a second career as a health coach in 2018, and developed a line of supplements that supposedly promote clear skin and shiny hair.[1] Although there is some research pointing to a connection between intestinal disorders like IBS and skin conditions like eczema—a link that researchers call the "gut-skin axis"—we're still a very long way from understanding why this connection exists, and whether it's a matter of correlation or causation.[2] It's possible (and I would say likely) that other factors—stress, poverty, underlying illness, and so on—could explain these disturbances in both the gut and the skin. To date there's no concrete evidence that healing gut issues will also heal the skin (though of course some people do have legitimate food allergies with symptoms like hives or rashes, which go away when they avoid the food), or that eating particular foods will lead to skin or gut healing.

That doesn't stop wellness culture from claiming otherwise.

"The best way to truly get your skin to glow from the inside out is by ensuring that you're eating a variety of superfoods," a 2019 *Healthline* article intones,[3] using a meaningless label that wellness media loves to slap on the latest trendy fruit or seed. But then, a few paragraphs later, the piece goes on to recommend various masks, facial oils, and serums—because "only the very best products revitalize your skin from the inside out, so it's worth investing in those you know will penetrate the skin and get to work from the inside out!"

The mental contortions required by that sentence belie one of wellness culture's dirty truths: "Glowing from within" actually means "putting a bunch of shit on your skin." Not just *on*, actually—sometimes it's *in*, as Gwyneth Paltrow can attest. The poster girl for wellness glow—who sells a variety of pricey face creams and exfoliants under her GOOPGLOW line—is open about the fact that even though she uses fancy skin care products and makes sure to "hydrate" (aka drinking water, another wellness-culture obsession), "sometimes a girl needs a little extra help" in the form of anti-wrinkle injectables. In a 2020 Instagram post, she announced a partnership with an injectable brand that she said helped her get rid of frown lines (and stayed on-brand by claiming that the product was "uniquely purified").[4] She's talked about other invasive facial treatments, too, including getting injected with her own platelets and having her face stung by bees.[5]

People generally lose fullness and elasticity in their skin as they age. The natural aging process means that after the age of twenty, the average person produces 1 percent less collagen in the skin each year.[6] And yet wellness culture, which typically lionizes all things "natural," isn't content to let nature take its course when it comes to aging. Instead, it pushes "age reversal." One of the latest trendy products marketed for that purpose is supplemental collagen, which is touted as having supposed benefits for numerous body systems, even though the main focus is cosmetic. Supplement companies promise that collagen will give you not only young, dewy skin and strong nails, but also strong bones, pain-free joints, and better digestion, though those claims aren't supported by sound evidence, or in some cases *any* evidence. And the health claims are really just a cover for the fact that this is a product that preys on people's (especially women's) societally conditioned fear of aging.

This is just another example of how wellness culture is intertwined with other harmful belief systems, such as diet culture and beauty culture, that are rooted in other forms of oppression. A beauty ideal that punishes women and femmes for aging serves to uphold patriarchy by detracting from the power and wisdom that naturally tend to accrue with age, undercutting people's self-esteem and damaging true well-being. This effect compounds the further away you get from conventional beauty standards.

None of this is meant to shame anyone for buying anti-aging products, which I've done myself, too—it's the culture and its relentless lionization of youth that's the problem. Many people feel they have no choice but to play the anti-aging game in order to get treated with the respect and dignity they deserve. Even Paltrow is a victim of this cultural pressure. Of course she's also adding to that pressure by framing "age-reversal" treatments as a necessary part of wellness (and profiting from the anti-aging products she sells), but she's still just as caught up in it as the rest of us—and perhaps even more so, since celebrities like her are constantly being scrutinized by the media.

Paltrow has also been a major promoter (and arguably an originator) of the "clean beauty" trend, which in some cases seems like a good thing. Many "clean" beauty products label themselves as cruelty-free and more environmentally friendly than their conventional counterparts. But in the beauty world, things are not always as they seem on the surface.

Despite the moralizing language, some "clean" products may not be any better than the conventional stuff. That's because the term "clean" is as meaningless as "superfoods"—since neither label is regulated, manufacturers can pretty much use them on anything. And that can lead to some rather unfortunate unintended consequences. People often have or develop allergies to "natural" ingredients like chamomile, lavender, and goat's milk found in "clean beauty" products.[7] For people with clinical skin conditions, like me, the wellness world's approach to skin care is often exclusionary—even as it pretends to cater to us with formulations that label themselves as treating eczema or calming sensitive skin. Essential oils and plant-based products can cause contact allergies and aggravate acne, further exacerbating the clinical conditions that they supposedly treat.

Part of the appeal of "clean beauty" is the aesthetic: packaging and design with lots of white space, soft colors, and powdery finishes. That look extends to all corners of the wellness industry, including blogs, books, and home design. "The pictures have this very particular look that are gorgeous and glistening and like everything seems like it's light and full of life," says Dawn Serra, describing one of the reasons she felt drawn to "clean eating" cookbooks and blogs.

The combination of open space and soft, floral hues presents a refreshing contrast to the fluorescent lights of offices and the clutter of work-from-home spaces where so many of us spend our days. The wellness aesthetic—part of an overarching millennial aesthetic that can now be found in the branding and packaging of many different industries—is all soft colors, daylight, houseplants, and calculated whimsy within a structure of cleanliness, orderliness. It's the free space we wish we had in our minds, a visual antidote to the emotional chaos of modern life.

Ironically, this very aspect of the wellness aesthetic also helps it play well on social media platforms, the source of much of that chaos. White space and muted, matte colors translate well to two-dimensional images on flat screens, notes writer Molly Fischer in *New York* magazine.[8] These images don't take as much work for the eye to parse in a quick scroll as do cluttered photos with saturated colors. And legibility on a phone screen is a primary—if not *the* primary—goal of millennial design. "*Instagrammable* is a term that does not mean 'beautiful' or even quite 'photogenic'; it means something more like 'readable,'" Fischer writes.

Another important aspect of the wellness aesthetic is that it also subtly evokes wealth. "Who can afford to have a space big enough that there's lots of empty space?" Serra says. "And who can afford to have, you know, floor to ceiling windows and fresh garden produce all the time?" An age-old trick of aspirational marketing is to get people to associate your product with wealth and beauty, by pairing it in ads with luxurious locations and conventionally attractive models. The wellness aesthetic does that for everything from workout clothes to period products, except instead of, say, the gilded trimmings of Trump Tower, its location-based markers of wealth are soft pastel backgrounds and uncluttered kitchens. Real walls and kitchens are marred by the splashes and scuffs of daily life, but the ones in the images used to sell wellness culture are kept pristine by the unseen hands of set designers and art directors.

Predictably, in reaction to all of this, a new trend has started to emerge in some corners of social media: "anti-aesthetic wellness." Still very much a part of wellness culture, anti-aesthetic wellness is Gen Z's tongue-in-cheek answer to the millennial brand of wellness that, as I write this, continues to dominate the space. Whereas the wellness aesthetic serves as a balm to the Internet-addled brain, anti-aesthetic wellness deliberately aggravates it. Anti-aesthetic wellness memes are intentionally ugly, with clashing colors and blurry SpongeBob screenshots covered in text like "fuck therapy i need to double dose on ashwagandha" and "when you get to the dust at the bottom of your adaptogenic latte." Both of these are from the Instagram meme page @seamossgirlies—arguably the progenitor of anti-aesthetic wellness—which its Gen-Z influencer founders launched "to break through the picture-perfect, aesthetic BS in wellness culture" while also serving an audience of "health / wellness weirdos" who love supplements, the gut microbiome, and other wellness-culture mainstays.

It remains to be seen whether anti-aesthetic wellness will catch on; for now it feels like more of a micro-trend, and a fun diversion from the current wellness landscape for people in the know. Yet the major issues with wellness culture go beyond just its aesthetic and how it reinforces unattainable, exclusionary standards of beauty and health. Indeed, one of these issues is the supplement industry itself, which unfortunately no version of wellness culture is calling out like it should.

### The Supplement Industry

When I was growing up, my family had an entire kitchen cabinet devoted to over-the-counter medications of various kinds. There was a colorful array of cold medicines and analgesics, antacids and ear drops, most of which were expired from lack of use. But scattered between the sticky bottles of cough suppressant and half-empty blister packs of antihistamines were the herbal and dietary supplements, and those saw a lot more action. When we felt even the slightest tickle in our throats, we downed vitamin C, zinc, and echinacea. If we had dry skin or hair, we popped vitamin E and flaxseed oil. My mom took big, chalky-looking pills filled with some kind of animal cartilage for a chronic knee injury, but they were there for the taking anytime my sister or I had a twinge of joint pain. As a teenager I chomped calcium chews designed for postmenopausal women. A daily multivitamin was de rigueur.

I continued using supplements as an adult, and never thought much about it until I started studying to become a dietitian and learned that except in the case of deficiencies or in certain special populations (for instance, people who are pregnant or breastfeeding), vitamin and mineral supplements generally aren't necessary. In fact, the vast majority of supplements don't have any demonstrable benefit. A 2022 review of eighty-four studies of vitamin and mineral supplements in more than seven hundred thousand participants found insufficient evidence that these supplements prevented cancer, cardiovascular disease, or death.[9] Some supplements may even *increase* the risk for certain diseases and overall mortality. Vitamin E, for example, was once thought to reduce the risk of heart disease, but then a few randomized controlled trials found that people who took vitamin E supplements actually had an increased risk of heart failure and death.[10] A similar thing happened with prostate cancer, where a randomized controlled trial of nearly thirty-five thousand men found that taking vitamin E supplements actually significantly raised their risk of getting the disease.[11] Meanwhile, a 2020 systematic review of the evidence (one of the best sources of scientific information) found that vitamin C increases the risk of lung cancer in women.[12] Despite what wellness culture would have you believe, supplements aren't a panacea—in fact they're quite the opposite in many cases. At best, they'll likely just give you what's often referred to as "expensive pee."

What's even more concerning is that most supplements are never independently tested for safety or efficacy, and in the U.S. there's no requirement that they be tested at all before going to market. Enforcement is hit-and-miss even if regulators do find problems. For example, the FDA documented in 2013 that nine weight-loss supplements on the market contained an amphetamine-like stimulant called beta-methylphenylethylamine (BMPEA), but two years later it still hadn't recalled those products or even publicly named them, according to a 2015 report by the *New York Times*.[13] It was only after the *Times* article was published that the FDA sent public warning letters to the companies responsible. Yet a 2021 study found nine banned and unapproved stimulant drugs—including BMPEA—in sports and weight-loss supplements then for sale in the U.S.[14] The warning letters had apparently had very little effect. Twenty percent of medication-related liver injury in the U.S. has been attributed to herbal and dietary supplements,[15] and one study found that supplements contribute to twenty-three thousand emergency room visits every year, with more than two thousand of those people (9 percent) going on to be hospitalized.[16] "The average consumer is just assuming that because it's in a bottle and it's sold in a store, somebody is a watchdog," said Catherine Price, journalist and author of *Vitamania*, in a 2020 podcast interview for *The Dream*.[17] "In the case of dietary supplement products...I just think it's very dangerous to assume that anyone's looking out for your health or safety."

Wellness culture talks a lot about "Big Pharma," which has its own problems, to be sure. But "Big Supplement" is arguably even more problematic because it's largely unregulated—the Wild West of medications. And it is indeed big business: the U.S. supplement industry was worth an estimated $37.2 billion in 2022, and the global market for nutritional supplements has reached an estimated $158 billion in 2023.[18] Yet in wellness culture, supplements are seen as being more natural and therefore better than medications, and many practitioners of complementary, integrative, and functional medicine prescribe supplements liberally.

Why does the supplement industry get away with only the barest of regulations, and why isn't there more outrage about that? A look at the history of the industry can help offer some answers. It all started around the turn of the twentieth century, the heyday of "patent medicines" in the U.S.

Popular throughout the 1800s, patent medicines were proprietary tonics and tinctures, potions and pills, that were marketed as cures for a wide variety of ailments. (Most manufacturers didn't actually have patents for their formulas, and many were very similar despite being sold under different labels.) Some patent-medicine marketers made claims that were more or less limited to one system of the body—digestive, respiratory, "female complaints"—but numerous others made outrageously overblown promises, like the nostrum that claimed to relieve "every ailment known to man, woman, and child."[19] Occasionally some of the ingredients in patent medicines had genuine medical value for certain ailments (quinine for malaria, digitalis for heart failure), but generally neither manufacturers nor buyers had the medical knowledge to administer the correct doses for the appropriate conditions. Instead, they were prescribed willy-nilly for every condition under the sun. What's more, numerous patent medicines were merely placebos, consisting of nothing more than sugar water and flavorings. Many of these supposed remedies also contained alcohol and/or harder drugs, including addictive ones like morphine, cocaine, or opium, which likely helped relieve pain and may have *felt* like they had other benefits, even if their primary effect was to make the user high (and often hooked, too).

Patent medicines were often marketed to women, and they were successful in part because at the time healthcare for women—not to mention Black and other marginalized people—was so lacking. Back then most doctors were men (the overwhelming majority of whom were white), and the patriarchal norms of the day meant that women were supposed to be modest and proper—not to talk openly about their bodies, and certainly not with men.[20] This meant that many women didn't feel comfortable discussing important issues like menstruation, fertility, pregnancy, abortion, childbirth, postpartum depression, or menopause with their doctors (if they were fortunate enough to even have access to doctors, which many did not, particularly in rural areas). Patent medicines stepped into that vacuum, offering the privacy and convenience of being available by mail order, and the promise of being able to address issues that were too embarrassing or poorly understood to discuss with doctors. In some ways, the patent-medicine industry was to women of the nineteenth century what Internet message boards and social media are to those of the twenty-first.

Unfortunately (as is often the case with online health advice today) patent medicines were largely ineffective and harmful, and the producers and sellers of patent medicines weren't exactly scrupulous. By the turn of the 20th century, some people were starting to get wise to that fact—one of whom was Samuel Hopkins Adams, an editor at *Collier's* magazine. He embarked on an ambitious investigative-reporting project that culminated in a 1905 series of articles exposing patent medicines as "The Great American Fraud."[21] The series called out nostrums like Peruna, which was the most popular patent medicine in the country at the time, claiming to cure a huge range of conditions including bunions, dyspepsia, heat rash, fever, and tuberculosis, to prevent hair loss, smallpox, sunstroke, nearsightedness, and to help arrest or reverse old age. Adams's investigation found that none of the drugs in Peruna were concentrated enough to produce any beneficial effect, which was true for a number of other patent medicines as well. The only truly "active" ingredient in many of these supposed remedies (including Peruna) was alcohol, though some also contained cocaine and opium. Adams reported 23 deaths attributable to acetanilide, an analgesic ingredient in many patent medicines including Peruna.

The articles were read by tens of thousands of people, including a number of lawmakers, who began crafting a bill to stop the patent-medicine menace. Soon thereafter, Upton Sinclair published *The Jungle*, which exposed the dirty underbelly of the American meat-processing industry. The book was a sensation, creating massive public demand for oversight of the nation's food production. Initially it seemed the government might side with the industry and sue Sinclair for libel on its behalf—until it began investigating his claims and found that the reality was, if anything, even worse than Sinclair had reported. In 1906, Congress passed the Pure Food and Drug Act, preventing food and drug manufacturers from making false statements on their labels, and requiring that drugs meet purity standards established by the United States Pharmacopeia, or the National Formulary.[22] The law defined "misbranding" and "adulteration" for the first time in a federal statute, and it prescribed penalties for each. It also established a federal regulatory organization (which later came to be known as the FDA) to monitor and enforce the new requirements.

Patent-medicine-industry lobbying eventually removed some of the Pure Food and Drug Act's bite, but the statute was still quite impactful. It required that ingredients deemed as "addictive" or "dangerous"—such as alcohol, morphine, and opium— be listed on the label if they were present. This truth-in-labeling law raised standards in the food and drug industries to protect consumers and helped put a stop to the shadier tactics of the patent-medicine trade. The Pure Food and Drug Act did have one major loophole that was revealed in a 1911 Supreme Court ruling, which said the law could only prohibit false and misleading statements about the *contents* of a drug, not about its therapeutic effects. But Congress quickly closed that loophole with the 1912 Sherley Amendment, which prohibited drug manufacturers from putting false therapeutic claims on their products' labels.

Meanwhile, in the early 1900s vitamins were beginning to be discovered, and by the 1920s the public was interested enough in vitamins that a new industry emerged to sell them. Vitamins, minerals, and other dietary supplements began to rise in popularity, just as regulations started to become more stringent. In 1930, Congress transferred enforcement duties to the newly named Food and Drug Administration, and eight years later it passed the Federal Food, Drug, and Cosmetic Act, which contained even more rigorous provisions, including requiring new drugs to be shown safe before marketing, and eliminating an amendment that had required drug misbranding cases prove "intent to defraud."

Naturally, makers of drugs and dietary supplements weren't too pleased with these requirements—and they began to push back. Although there were numerous other amendments to the law over the years, the first fatal blow to the FDA's power to regulate dietary supplements came in 1976. In the 1960s and 1970s, in the face of a ballooning market for foods and other products with added vitamins and minerals, the FDA had proposed new rules to combat public confusion about supplements and protect consumers from vitamin overdoses. The agency attempted to ensure that products with added vitamins and minerals could only include a maximum of 150 percent of the recommended daily allowance; otherwise, these products would (quite reasonably, I'd say) be classified as drugs.[23] The FDA also had tried to standardize supplement strengths and restrict the number of combinations of vitamins and minerals that could be sold.

In response, the industry's lobbying machine went into overdrive, organizing a major letter-writing campaign to pressure members of Congress to stop regulating supplements.[24] To get consumers on board with the campaign, industry groups argued that any attempt by the FDA to regulate supplements would be an infringement on personal freedom—a powerful goad for a certain subset of Americans.

The consumer-freedom argument worked, and the industry succeeded in getting scores of angry letters delivered to Congress. As a result, in 1976, Congress passed the Rogers-Proxmire Amendment (often known simply as the Proxmire Amendment), which effectively prevented the FDA from setting limits on the contents of supplements. It made it illegal for the FDA to create standards for supplements, classify them as drugs, or even require that they only contain ingredients with demonstrated benefits. The amendment also forbade the FDA from limiting the quantity of vitamins/minerals or the number of different ingredients that a supplement could contain, unless the agency could provide solid evidence that the product was unsafe. Essentially it put the burden of proof on the FDA rather than on supplement manufacturers. Alexander Schmidt, the FDA commissioner at the time, said the amendment was a "charlatan's dream." The market for dietary supplements exploded after Proxmire took effect: what was a $500 million industry in 1971 grew to $2 billion within ten years and $3 billion by 1988.[25]

The amendment forced the FDA to back off from regulating supplements' contents, but it didn't end the fight—far from it. In the late 1980s and early 1990s, supplement companies were starting to make more and more far-fetched claims about their products; in response, the FDA proposed regulations on the kinds of health claims that could be made on food package labels, product inserts, and store displays. Though the proposed rules actually allowed more leeway for claims on some food product labels, they likely also would have prevented most vitamin makers from saying that their products prevented disease and promoted health. Then, in the early 1990s, based on new evidence of harm from megadoses of vitamins and amino acids, the FDA released a proposal arguing that vitamins and minerals should have limited doses, that amino acids were not legal in supplements, and that herbal products are "inherently therapeutic" and therefore shouldn't be sold as dietary supplements, but instead treated as drugs (again quite reasonably, in my opinion).

The combination of these proposed regulations caused a panic in the supplement industry, which began to push for even stronger legal protections.

It enlisted the support of two unlikely allies: Democratic senator Tom Harkin and Republican senator Orrin Hatch. Though bipartisan support for anything was hard to come by even back then, these two senators had interests in common. In the early 1990s, Harkin became a convert to alternative medicine, after having claimed to have cured his allergies using bee pollen.[26] He also happened to be the person in charge of the budget for the National Institutes of Health (NIH), and he harnessed the position to champion the alt-med cause, using nearly a fifth of the agency's budget to establish the National Center for Complementary and Alternative Medicine (later renamed the National Center for Complementary and Integrative Health,[27] in an apparent effort to distance it from alternative medicine). Hatch, for his part, also claimed that bee pollen had cured his allergies. Hatch's home state of Utah was (and is) home to many alternative-medicine and dietary-supplement companies—the supplement industry was Utah's third-largest industry at the time (now it's the largest)—and of course those companies' bottom line would be hampered by FDA regulation, which Hatch, as a major recipient of supplement-industry campaign contributions, had an interest in preventing.[28]

So in 1994, Hatch and Harkin drafted the Dietary Supplement Health and Education Act (DSHEA), aimed at curtailing the FDA's power to regulate supplements.[29]

The law passed unanimously, thanks in large part to lobbying by supplement-industry groups that relied heavily on the old government-wants-to-limit-your-freedom argument. In one particularly memorable ad created by a supplement lobbying group in 1993, a SWAT team enters a house and storms into the bathroom of a flustered Mel Gibson, who, holding a bottle in his outstretched hands, shouts "Hey, guys…guys, it's only vitamins! Vitamin C—you know, like in oranges?" Then, in voice-over, with white text on a black background: "If you don't want to lose your vitamins, make the FDA stop. Call the U.S. Senate and tell them that you want to take your vitamins in peace. If enough of us do that, it'll work."[30] It did work, resulting in more letters to Congress than were received about the Vietnam War.

DSHEA virtually eliminated the government's ability to regulate the supplement industry. It made it so that the FDA no longer had any authority to block supplements from going to market; instead, the agency could only take action after the fact if it learned of health and safety issues with a given product. DSHEA also defined supplements much more broadly than they'd been defined before, to include not only vitamins and minerals, but also herbal and botanical products, amino acids, other dietary substances, and derivatives, extracts, or combinations of these ingredients. Before DSHEA, the FDA had proposed regulating herbs as drugs because of their potency—some herbal preparations can be even stronger than pharmaceuticals. But because of DSHEA, there's no upper limit on the dosage of herbal supplements.

What's more, manufacturers were now allowed to make unproven claims about their products' effects on the "structure or function" of the body (even though they were still prohibited from making outright promises to treat or prevent disease). The "structure/function" loophole is why supplements can say things like "supports a healthy immune system" or "improves gastrointestinal health," which may suggest, to unwitting consumers, that the products' reach is infinite—that supplements can ward off acute illnesses like COVID or chronic ones like IBS, even if the manufacturers don't come out and say that directly.

In early 2022, the FDA proposed amending DSHEA to require that basic information about each supplement product be listed annually with the agency, so that it could more quickly identify and take action against dangerous or illegal products on the market. Predictably, some within the industry are opposed to such a listing requirement, and as of this writing it remains simply a proposal.

Meanwhile, the market for supplements is booming. The fact that these products legally *aren't allowed* to undergo the rigorous and lengthy FDA testing process that drugs do before becoming available to consumers means that supplement companies can churn out new products as they like. And the major players in the global supplement industry include well-known pharmaceutical and multilevel marketing companies (MLMs)—Pfizer, Amway (Nutrilite), Bayer AG, Abbott Laboratories, GSK, Archer Daniels Midland, and Herbalife International, among others—giving the lie to the notion that dietary supplements are somehow completely separate from and more "natural" than pharmaceuticals.

Knowing all of this, I have a very different relationship with supplements today than I did when I was growing up. I'm far warier of supplements than I am of either pharmaceuticals or over-the-counter medications, both of which are required by the FDA to be established as safe and effective before going to market. I no longer believe that supplements are harmless by virtue of being "natural," and in fact I'm careful to avoid added herbs, vitamins, and minerals lest they interact with my thyroid medication or aggravate my autoimmune conditions. Normally I don't take any supplements unless bloodwork shows a deficiency (like the anemia I had during pregnancy), but as I write this I have a nine-month-old baby who is breastfeeding, so I'm still taking a prenatal multivitamin and some additional vitamin D as recommended by my doctor and lactation consultant. I have a few shelves in my own home devoted to over-the-counter drugs, and scattered among the cold medicines and cough drops are a few bottles of vitamin B6—which I took for nausea early in my pregnancy—that are now expired.

### Cultural Appropriation

Each year, as many as twenty thousand Western tourists journey to the remote Amazonian city of Iquitos—reachable only by air or boat—to drink ayahuasca, a hallucinogenic brew made from a blend of local plants that are believed to have healing properties in addition to—and in many cases because of—their psychedelic ones.[31] Tourists attend ostensibly traditional ayahuasca healing ceremonies to take "the Medicine" and experience powerful hallucinations that some credit with saving their lives.

But according to ethnographer and journalist Carlos Suárez Álvarez, who studies the contemporary culture of ayahuasca in the Amazon, there's nothing traditional about these ceremonies.[32] In local Indigenous healing traditions, he explained in the 2020 Netflix docuseries *(Un)well*, it's often only the *healer* who drinks the ayahuasca (known as *yagé* in some Amazonian Indigenous communities[33]), using it to channel different energies to their patients in chants or songs. "These songs are the medicine," Álvarez said—not the ayahuasca itself. The people who run Iquitos's ayahuasca lodges are often foreigners who are disconnected from the Indigenous roots of these ceremonies. They're appropriating ayahuasca from the cultures that depend on it, depleting the plant and creating shortages in the local area—and yet Westerners may not recognize this appropriation, believing the lodge-based ceremonies to be "authentic." As Álvarez bluntly puts it, for Western tourists, "you will never get a traditional ayahuasca treatment."

The appropriation of ayahuasca by lodges catering to tourists is driven by many factors, including economic forces and, among the clients, a genuine need for healing. But a major driver of this and many other forms of cultural appropriation that are rampant in wellness culture is the same belief we've been discussing throughout this chapter: that "natural" is always better. In this view, non-Western forms of medicine are seen as being "ancient" and traditional, unsullied by the hand of the medical-industrial complex and Big Pharma, and therefore natural and good. The truth is often not that simple, because when traditional healing practices get cut off from their roots and commodified for a Western audience, they can cause significant harm.

Ayahuasca, for example, can be extremely dangerous for the

tourists at the lodges. Westerners who attend ayahuasca ceremonies are often suffering and seeking relief from serious issues: trauma and PTSD, depression, anxiety, chronic pain. For people who have existing mental-health issues, and especially for those who are on psychotropic medications, taking ayahuasca may cause complications including seizures and psychotic episodes. Even without these extreme side effects, taking ayahuasca is largely unpleasant for many people and can result in symptoms such as vomiting, diarrhea, high blood pressure, elevated heart rate, anxiety, and paranoia. The lodges don't always do a great job of checking people's mental-health background, and tourists also sometimes lie or conceal the truth about their conditions because they're so desperate for help. They've been told that the visions produced by ayahuasca will set them free. And yet the traditional brews don't always produce visions. So, under pressure to give their customers what they want, some ayahuasca lodges add another hallucinogenic plant to the usual blend to more reliably induce hallucinations — but with dangerous potential side effects like heart attacks and death.

Some people — including both Western visitors and locals — feel that ayahuasca saves lives, and that it should be available to everyone who wants it. Psychedelics including ayahuasca have become popular for treating trauma and other conditions (including, in some cases, eating disorders) in pockets of the psychotherapy world, backed by some promising early-stage scientific research. I personally know people who've had numerous positive experiences taking ayahuasca and other psychedelics. Some people also believe that the ayahuasca tourism industry is helping to improve economic conditions for people in lower-income countries in the global South.

Yet a group of Indigenous leaders in the Amazon who specialize in ayahuasca medicine argue that it's dangerous on many levels for ayahuasca to be used outside of its traditional context, and these are the voices that should matter most in this discussion. According to Miguel Evanjuanoy Chindoy, an Indigenous-rights activist in Putumayo, Colombia, and a spokesperson for the Union of Indigenous Yagé Medics of the Colombian Amazon (UMIYAC), "the level of cultural appropriation that is being conducted by outsiders—tourists, organizations that come in wanting to research and medicalize this plant—is very preoccupying for a people that has been struggling to protect their territory."[34] He explained through a translator in a 2020 webinar that in local Indigenous communities, medicinal plants like those used to make ayahuasca are seen as a form of collective knowledge—but Westerners are coming in and treating these plants as a form of property, which is impacting the community's notions of collective ownership in concerning ways. Instead of sharing the benefits of the plants freely within the community, some people are now selling these plants to the outside world for profit, enriching themselves at the expense of the community. Indeed, Álvarez estimates that the ayahuasca lodges in Iquitos alone bring in millions of dollars per year.[35]

Chindoy says there are some young Indigenous people from the Amazon who hold themselves out as traditional healers despite not having a full understanding of the *yagé* plant. As a group of UMIYAC members and other Indigenous Amazonian political and spiritual leaders wrote in a 2019 joint declaration on cultural appropriation, these faux healers "disguise themselves with feathers and necklaces and call themselves *taitas*, a general term of respect commonly used in communities of the Inga people [of Colombia]. The goal of these practitioners is to seek profit."[36] These ersatz *taitas* typically leave home and go into the cities or abroad to ply their trade, to the detriment of both the Indigenous communities and the unsuspecting tourists who pay them. "Not having real spiritual knowledge, they put the mental, physical and spiritual health and even the lives of their own patients at risk," the declaration states. It also calls out the non-Indigenous people who "appropriate and abuse our practices" by holding ayahuasca ceremonies, leading spiritual retreats, and operating shamanism schools.

In the 2020 webinar, a participant asked how one might work with ayahuasca in the United States while respecting Indigenous communities. "I've had many conversations with the elders about this, and this medicine needs to remain anchored to its endemic place," Chindoy said. To anyone who wants to take ayahuasca out of the Amazon and bring it to Western countries, he recommended reflecting deeply on why they would want to do this. The joint declaration on cultural appropriation puts it more bluntly: "No one outside the indigenous communities can cultivate, sell *yagé* or officiate ceremonies. According to our own customary systems, the only people who can perform *yagé* ceremonies are the [healers] who have the endorsement and the recognition of the Amazonian indigenous communities, of our traditional authorities and of Indigenous organizations such as UMIYAC."

Ayahuasca is just one of many healing traditions that have come under threat in this way. Countless others have been taken from cultures around the world, and then whitewashed and sold to mainstream Western audiences under the banner of wellness. In the process, wellness culture is both twisting these traditional practices beyond recognition, and often irreparably damaging the communities that rely on them.

Cultural appropriation in the wellness world is often tied to orientalism — simplistic, inaccurate Western ideas about Asian and Middle Eastern cultures that portray them as mysterious, never changing, and (in the case of wellness) possessed of some mystical healing knowledge that Westerners can extract and own. As writer Kylie Cheung noted in *Salon*, the 2021 Hulu series *Nine Perfect Strangers* epitomizes the orientalism of the wellness industry.[37] The show stars Nicole Kidman as ethereal wellness guru Masha Dmitrichenko, who owns an idyllic yet eerie retreat center called Tranquillum that's filled with natural beauty and gives rise to the occasional ghost sighting. The setting looks like it was lifted straight off a wellness influencer's Instagram page, with peaceful woods, waterfalls, and hot springs—as well as many Asian-inflected trappings such as meditation and acupuncture practices, white robes that vaguely resemble the attire of Buddhist monks, and gongs and other Asian-inspired decor. These tropes are so common in wellness spaces that they may not even register as orientalist or appropriated from another culture—in their very ubiquity lies the damage they cause. The wellness industry uses elements of Asian cultures to create a calming vibe and spaces that are sometimes genuinely healing to the people who come to them—and yet the industry, rather than the appropriated cultures, is what benefits most. "It's often mystical white women like Masha who are cashing in on the West's fetishization of eastern culture and spirituality," Cheung writes.

This disconnect is strikingly evident in the yoga world, where capitalism has obscured the practice's real roots. Susanna Barkataki, a yoga teacher trainer, author, and advocate for diversity, equity, and inclusion in yoga, explains that yoga is a spiritual practice that has at least eight different tenets or "limbs." These limbs, which are meant to be practiced in progression, include ethical principles for treating others and the world (called the *yamas*), standards of personal behavior (called *niyamas*), physical postures (*asana*), breathwork (*pranayama*), sensory focus (*pratyahara*), concentration or single-pointed focus (*dharana*), meditation (*dhyana*), and finally liberation (*samadhi*).[38] The physical practice is merely one aspect of yoga, and it's a pretty early step on the path to liberation.

"Most of what we see in Western yoga spaces or wellness spaces is really just focused on a misunderstanding of *asana*, of one of the eight limbs," Barkataki says. "And so this kind of bodily focused, fitness-focused illusion of what yoga is—like 'yoga is wellness,' or 'yoga will teach you to be thin and healthy and always, always happy'—none of that is really what the focus of yoga is. It was a spiritual practice to help alleviate suffering and aimed at personal and collective liberation."

Barkataki says that "workout yoga classes" really miss the point, as does the commodification of the symbols and language of yoga. When words like *om* and *namaste* are taken out of context and plastered on yoga mats or T-shirts, it's blatant cultural appropriation that exemplifies the Western impulse to cherry-pick the parts of yoga we want and leave the rest—the colonizing element at the heart of the Western relationship with yoga. And when yoga is presented simply as an exercise regimen, it leaves out many important aspects of the practice that could have real benefits for both individual and collective well-being. "There is this system for freedom, for liberation, and we could be taking part or sharing or teaching or practicing more of that, and we're not," she says.

Barkataki, who is of Indian and British descent, doesn't say that only people of South Asian heritage should practice or teach yoga. "Yoga is a practice of unity, and so it really is available to everyone," she says. "Any race or religion, we can all benefit from yoga as a path to bring us more peace and more freedom." She encourages everyone who practices yoga to go deeper into the practice over time, so that they're not just staying stuck in the surface-level, wellness-culture version of yoga. She also urges practitioners to ask teachers to make their classes more accessible to people with a wider range of bodies and backgrounds. As for those teachers, Barkataki says that great yoga instructors can come from all different backgrounds— and that in order to avoid being appropriative, teachers can learn to teach yoga in a way that truly honors the tradition it comes from. For teachers who aren't Indian or South Asian, that means "decolonizing your bookshelves, reading texts from South Asian and Indian authors, reading *Yoga Sutras* translations from South Asian teachers, and taking classes from people from within the tradition who can share about it in a culturally competent and honoring and respectful way," she says. "Because it's those teachers who often are erased in the sight of their own wisdom traditions, and so centering those who've been left out [can help] to counter that oppression and omission."

This vision of yoga that includes people from diverse backgrounds without erasing its originators helps honor the communities where yoga was developed, while also acknowledging the deep hunger among Westerners and particularly Americans for practices that nurture the mind, body, and spirit. The Western belief system posits a split between mind and body, rational and emotional, individual and collective, and its American iteration lionizes not just the mind and the rational, but also the individual. American culture teaches us that our health is our own responsibility, that if we have a problem we need to bootstrap our way out of it rather than relying on collective care. In a culture like this, it's no wonder so many of us have felt lost and out of touch with our bodies. It's no wonder we have a healthcare system that makes so many people feel dismissed, unseen, cut off from their wholeness. It's no wonder so many people are interested in forms of medicine that purport to treat the whole person (whether or not they actually achieve that).

Currently, however, the way yoga is packaged and sold in wellness culture centers Westerners and excludes people from the communities that birthed the practice, as well as people of color more generally. That erasure is glaringly evident in mainstream media about yoga. In a 2019 study, sociologist Sabrina Strings and colleagues analyzed cover images and articles featured in *Yoga Journal* between 1975 and 2015. They found that since 1998—which they cite as the beginning of the latest yoga boom in the U.S., initially sparked by celebrities such as Madonna and Sting touting yoga not as a millennia-old holistic practice but as a regimen of body shrinking and sculpting—there's been a significant decline in the number of men and people of color on the magazine's covers.[39] Instead, full-body shots of white women have come to dominate the magazine's imagery, the researchers found. The articles, meanwhile, "promote yoga as a part of a beauty regime, [which] relies on a dubious mix of self-love and fat aversion for white women, while people of color are almost entirely excluded from consideration."

In framing yoga as a way for white women to "tame fat" while ignoring people of color, *Yoga Journal* is just one of many culprits. I remember that around 1999, when I was first exposed to yoga, a mainstream teen magazine published a series of poses meant to "tone the thighs"; they were demonstrated by an impossibly thin white woman. My then boyfriend, who was Indian American, reacted with disgust when I told him I was doing "thigh yoga," rightly pointing out that there's no such thing and that yoga is so much more than a workout routine, let alone one targeting a specific body part. I kept doing the poses for a while anyway, guiltily and in secret, already unconsciously compelled by the message that yoga was a way to make my body conform to the standards of white feminine beauty. In the decades since, countless media (and social media) portrayals have depicted yoga as a way to shrink the body and attain the extremely thin physique of white, self-styled wellness gurus like Nicole Kidman's Masha—even if the media in question don't explicitly come out and say the words "weight loss."

This thinness-focused version of yoga can perpetuate damaging stereotypes of Asian people and cultures. "As a yoga instructor, I have heard online coaches and fellow yogis encourage veganism (as a weight-loss initiative and not an environmental/ethical one) on the premise that Asian peoples' diets are typically plant-based, and most Asian people are thin," writes Ruth Flynn, a yoga teacher working toward a master's in medical anthropology at George Washington University.[40] "This is revealing itself in an ever-expanding story where West = fat and East = thin." Both of those equations can be damaging to people's self-image, obscuring the diversity of body sizes and shapes in the world, and preventing the acceptance of all bodies.

Diet culture is also prevalent in Western versions of Ayurveda—a form of traditional medicine from India (where it's regulated as a branch of "Indian medicine," as distinct from "modern medicine"[41]). Ayurveda emphasizes the integration of mind, body, and spirit, using practices including herbal remedies, exercise, meditation, breathing, and physical therapy as well as particular ways of eating. Ayurveda has become popular in some Western countries, where it tends to be sold as a diet—cut out this food for this condition, take this plant for that one, that sort of thing—and can be quite restrictive.

But according to Barkataki, who is also trained as an Ayurvedic practitioner, true Ayurveda isn't actually the diet-y regimen it's made out to be. She gives an example from her training, which included a practicum where students had to diagnose hypothetical patients and prescribe treatments for them. One of these patients was presented as having acid stomach, lots of anxiety, and difficulty sleeping, and they were said to be drinking eight cups of coffee a day and eating lots of spicy foods. Barkataki's group, probably like many students of Ayurveda in the West (and many dietitians and doctors, for that matter), jumped to a sweeping prescription: cut out coffee, cut out spicy food. "And our teacher just smiled and laughed and said, 'What I would tell them is drink seven cups of coffee a day and come back next week and let's talk,'" Barkataki says. "So it's a very different kind of targeted, individualized, gradual approach—it's not restrictive in the same way." She says that unfortunately many popular, recent books about Ayurveda—even some written by South Asian authors—present Ayurvedic dietary changes in a much more restrictive way. "That, I would say, is a misunderstanding of what Ayurveda is," she says.

Another misunderstanding has to do with how different herbs are prescribed in the Westernized versions of Ayurveda.

Barkataki explains that the philosophy is "very specifically oriented towards an individual person—it's not a one-size-fits-all approach." Ayurvedic practitioners don't, for example, prescribe the same herbs to everyone with a particular condition. And yet when Ayurveda gets transferred to the West, that's exactly what happens. Some naturopathic, integrative, and functional-medicine practitioners even have herb and supplement protocols that they recommend to *all* their patients, regardless of condition. "Particular herbs like ashwagandha or shatavari become these hot-button herbs, like, oh, everyone needs to do this for hormonal balance or whatever," Barkataki says. "But that's actually not true—that's not how an Ayurvedic practitioner or physician would ever recommend those herbs to be used. It's not a generalized approach." Once again, Western wellness culture distorts a traditional healing practice developed by people of color, taking the parts that fit with its worldview and discarding the rest.

This is part of the orientalist, colonizing tendency in wellness culture that views anything "ancient" and non-Western as good and seeks to co-opt and capitalize on it—but only certain parts. And that's often where it goes wrong, because when healing traditions are stripped down and divorced from the cultures and the value systems that they're a part of, can they really be called healing *traditions* anymore? Or do they simply become commodities, products to be bought and sold in a capitalistic system? When Western wellness practitioners offer yoga, Ayurveda, ayahuasca ceremonies, or any manner of other non-Western healing practices, often what they're actually selling is a simulacrum—the souvenir for tourists at the airport gift shop, the faux-traditional artifact devoid of meaning and context. It might still have some value for the people buying and selling it, but it can never come close to capturing the whole that it's been cut off from. The irony of framing these appropriated practices as part of a "holistic" approach to health is apparently lost on wellness culture.

Kimberly J. Lau, a professor of literature at the University of California at Santa Cruz who studies feminist theory, race, and popular culture, writes that this commodification has at its core "the belief in personal transformation through alternative, non-Western paradigms of health and wellness." As she explains in her book *New Age Capitalism*, "popular alternative health practices like aromatherapy, macrobiotic eating, yoga, tai chi, and their related products exploit their associations—both real and imagined—with global, non-Western cultures."[42] (The book was published in 2001, when the macrobiotic diet and tai chi were among the most popular wellness trends, but today a whole host of other culturally appropriative trends have taken their place.) Wellness culture tends to downplay the religious roots of many of non-Western practices, while also capitalizing on the hunger in Western culture for a kind of timeless spirituality that exists in contrast to the hard rationality of science and medicine.

Again, part of the reason that exploitation works is that Western medicine has real shortcomings, for which wellness culture frames so-called Eastern medicine as the cure. People with trauma, chronic illness, chronic pain, and other poorly understood conditions often don't find satisfying solutions in the conventional Western medical system. The fact that mainstream medical care doesn't generally address or even inquire about patients' mental, emotional, and spiritual lives can leave people feeling like alternative medicine has more to offer. It can lead physicians themselves to this conclusion, too, which may explain the rise in "integrative" and "functional" approaches that attempt to marry non-Western philosophies and conventional medicine.

Yet in the effort to address what's missing from the health-care system, these approaches are not only often appropriating and cherry-picking other cultures' healing traditions, but they're also overlooking a fundamentally important aspect of collective, population-level well-being: the social determinants of health, which we'll turn to next.

# CHAPTER 3

# Determinants

In February of 2020, as concerns over the novel coronavirus started to intensify, searches for phrases like "immune boost" and "immune boosting" began to surge.[1] People were clamoring for information about how to protect themselves, how to have some control in an increasingly uncertain situation. Health authorities like the CDC weren't doing a great job of communicating with the public, and wellness influencers, celebrities, and supplement peddlers moved quickly into that vacuum, offering recipes, food products, tonics, workouts, yoga poses, essential oils, and more to supposedly strengthen the immune system, with little to no evidence to support their claims. Questionable stem-cell clinics soon began marketing their treatments as a way to boost immunity against the virus, again without sound evidence.[2] As the pandemic wore on, even relatively mainstream health-media outlets and healthcare organizations got in on the act. A piece from *Medical Daily* reposted on MSN (Microsoft Network) promised "12 Best Immune Booster Vitamins & Supplements for COVID-19 and Flu."[3] On CNBC, a nutritionist shared her "5 Favorite Immunity-Boosting Recipes to Stay Healthy During Covid-19."[4]

In reality, there's no such thing as "immune boosting." The concept is misleading and scientifically inaccurate; the immune system is far more complex and multifaceted than wellness culture makes it out to be, and it can't simply be "boosted" by foods, supplements, herbs, and the like. Yet it's completely understandable why there would be a market for supposedly immune-boosting products during a global pandemic. In times of uncertainty about our health, when we're desperate for answers and for protection, wellness culture preys on our anxiety. Bogus wellness products and practices tend to proliferate in those situations, as they did throughout the pandemic. They succeed because they offer the illusion that we can have some control over our fate by taking supplements or doing certain yoga poses, rather than the much more difficult truth that we don't have much control as individuals, beyond taking basic precautions like mask-wearing, social distancing, and vaccination. Following wellness culture's dubious "immune-boosting" protocols makes it feel like you're taking your health into your own hands, but ultimately they don't do what they promise—and in some cases they even cause harm.

In fact, the pandemic has revealed how little individual control we really have over our health, and how much public health policy and socioeconomic factors actually determine our level of collective well-being. Of course we can reduce our personal risk by getting vaccinated and wearing masks indoors—proven strategies that unfortunately got denigrated and dismissed in certain overlapping circles of wellness culture and politics, as we'll discuss in the following chapters. And vaccination and masking are both public health measures, not just personal ones, since they affect more than just the individual.

But as far as population well-being is concerned, the most important factors are the ones wellness culture routinely ignores—those that are out of our individual control: the social determinants of health.

## Social Determinants of Health

Social determinants are the conditions under which people live, and the economic and social forces that shape our lives from birth and childhood through work, aging, and death. These determinants fall into five main categories, according to the CDC: healthcare access and quality; education access and quality; social and community context; economic stability; and neighborhood and built environment. At a more granular level, these determinants include income, food and housing security, experiences of discrimination, job security, exposure to air and water pollution, and many other social and environmental factors that influence our health risks and can contribute to worse outcomes for the marginalized. For example, being uninsured (or underinsured) can lead people to delay or skip necessary medical visits and forgo medications, potentially worsening their health over time. The same is true for weight stigma, which also can increase the risk of poor mental and physical health, as can exposure to community violence.[5] And racism is a social determinant of health that can both interact with and operate independently of other social determinants: a 2009 review of the evidence found that at equal levels of socioeconomic status, insurance coverage, and healthcare access, Americans of color still receive lower-quality medical care than white Americans.[6]

Diet and wellness culture would have you believe that health disparities largely come down to eating and exercise, and that they could be fixed if marginalized groups simply had the education and access needed to "eat healthy" and move more. And yes, nutrition and physical activity do play a role in health and can be impacted by poverty and lack of access; food apartheid, food insecurity, and neighborhood safety can all affect eating and activity levels.

But in reality, food and exercise are far less important for collective well-being than they're made out to be. Several studies have shown that, apart from genetics, what primarily determines the health of a population are social factors. About *70 percent* of health outcomes are attributable to socioeconomic factors, access to and quality of healthcare, and the physical environment. Only 10 percent of population health outcomes are attributable to diet and exercise combined.[7] The remaining 20 percent are attributable to behaviors such as smoking, alcohol and drug use, sexually transmitted diseases, and teen birth. In other words, the vast majority of factors affecting our collective well-being have nothing to do with food and exercise—or with individual behaviors at all—and everything to do with the conditions in which we live.

Living in wellness culture, it's understandable that many people believe the reverse—that the only things that really matter are nutrition, physical activity, and perhaps other pursuits like meditation or taking supplements, and that social and economic factors play a small role. But that simply isn't true, and wellness culture puts our well-being at risk by encouraging supposedly health-optimizing behaviors that have little benefit and great potential for harm. When someone is struggling with basic survival—the foundation of Maslow's hierarchy of needs—what good are juice cleanses or fitness classes or skin care? These things are wildly inaccessible for anyone in that situation, but even if they were within reach financially, spending time and energy on the pursuit of so-called wellness just isn't a long-term solution when the problem is deeper, rooted in systems beyond individual control.

All of this has played out in stark ways during the COVID-19 pandemic, a glaring example of how social determinants can profoundly affect people's risk of infection, severe illness, and death. Occupation is a social determinant: "essential workers" are at higher risk because they can't work from home, tend to work in settings that increase COVID exposure by putting them in frequent contact with other people, and often don't get paid sick leave. Income is another: lower-income people tend to lack access to quality healthcare and culturally competent care, putting them at risk of serious disease. The physical environment is yet another: air pollution in certain neighborhoods may increase people's chances of developing respiratory illnesses. And crowded housing is another still, making viral transmission more likely. No one determinant is entirely within individual control, and no number of "immune-boosting" products and practices could keep people from getting COVID when the systemic conditions of their lives are putting them in the path of the virus every single day.

The social determinants of health were originally recognized by public health scholars in the 1990s, well before the advent of social media, when the Internet was just a tiny fraction of the vast informational landscape that it is today. But in the decades since, access to online health information and exposure to misinformation have become increasingly prevalent, to the point where some researchers now argue that the *info-sphere*—the realm of data, information, knowledge, and communication—needs to be recognized as another social determinant of health, distinct from but intimately linked to socioeconomic, environmental, and cultural conditions.[8] The infosphere is the information environment in which people live, and in Western culture today it's largely digital. (Even the information reported in offline sources is shaped by input from the Internet and social media; Twitter often functions as the unofficial assignment desk of legacy media outlets.) And the online infosphere has had increasingly deleterious effects in recent years, especially during the pandemic. Like polluted air or contaminated water, online health mis- and disinformation are bringing disease in their wake—causing a steep rise in vaccine hesitancy that has led to the reemergence of vaccine-preventable diseases; discouraging people from seeking medical care for serious illnesses like cancer; promoting eating disorders and fad diets; and much more. Misinformation is now recognized as a major and far-ranging threat to public health, compounding the risk of many other diseases.

The infosphere intersects with other social determinants of

health, creating disproportionate impacts on those who are marginalized. Several studies have found that people with lower income levels and lower levels of education (a group in which Black and Hispanic people are overrepresented) are more likely to have relatively low levels of online health literacy—and that this, in turn, makes people more likely to use and trust dubious sources of health and wellness information, such as social media posts. In trying to judge whether a source of wellness information is credible, those with low online health literacy tend to take their cues from social proof—likes and shares, as well as celebrity endorsements and recommendations from friends— which they perceive as signals of trustworthiness, whereas they view health information from specialist doctors as being less trustworthy.[9]

Certainly there are reasons some people might distrust Western medical doctors other than low health literacy, including having had their symptoms dismissed or having been discriminated against in the healthcare system. Conventional medicine is subject to the same systemic biases—misogyny, racism, fatphobia, to name just a few—as every other field (including alternative medicine), and those can be enacted in the doctor's office in ways that are especially noxious given the intimacy of the healthcare setting.

Indeed, it's not just access to care that contributes to people's health outcomes, but also the quality of that care. And for too many people—particularly those who are already marginalized in some way—healthcare quality is sorely lacking. For example, research has consistently shown that Black patients are systematically undertreated for pain relative to white patients, and a 2016 study of medical students and residents found that 50 percent of participants endorsed at least one false and racist belief such as "Black people's nerve endings are less sensitive than white people's," "Black people's skin is thicker than white people's," and "Black people's blood coagulates more quickly than white people's."[10] When patients aren't given the opportunity to explain their own pain and are instead subjected to harmful racial stereotypes, it's bound to take a toll on their relationship with the healthcare system.

These issues have historical roots in the British slave trade. During that moment in history, there was a major shift in the understanding of sickness and disease that led to corresponding changes in the doctor-patient relationship, says Carolyn Roberts, a historian of medicine and science at Yale University who is working on a book called *To Heal and to Harm: Medicine, Knowledge, and Power in the British Slave Trade.* In Britain and across Europe, diseases were starting to be understood not as imbalances in bodily fluids (the "four humors" of blood, phlegm, black bile, and yellow bile), as they previously had been, but rather as properties of organs and tissues. When the humoral theory was dominant, "patient self-reporting was absolutely crucial to the clinical encounter," Roberts told me in an email. But when the focus shifted to organs and tissues, doctors' technical knowledge of anatomy and how disease affected the body began to supplant people's reports of their own experience. "The patient's narrative began to disappear, and patients' experiential knowledge of their illness held little space in the clinical encounter," Roberts says.

That lack of space for patients' subjective understanding and the view that providers' knowledge is paramount still often play out today in Western medicine, in ways that can both negatively affect people's health and drive them to wellness-culture practices that in some cases cause further harm. Alternative medicine is frequently framed as doing a better job of listening and responding to people's self-reports, and indeed that's often the case; providers in those spaces tend to have more time and empathy for patients, which can have a positive impact (called the care effect) even if their prescriptions or recommendations themselves aren't effective. Yet a dismissive provider-patient dynamic also frequently shows up in alternative and integrative medicine, where the patient's narrative (for example, "cutting out food doesn't seem to be helping") can get brushed aside in favor of the provider's assessment ("food is definitely causing your health problems").

In considering the social determinants of health, the fact that the sometimes contentious relationship between health-care providers and patients emerged in part with the slave trade can't be ignored. In fact, Roberts argues, slave ships and the institution of slavery in general were central to the development and modernization of Western medicine. "On the slave ship, doctors were committing violence against enslaved people in order to keep them alive, brutalizing them in ways that went way beyond what was going on in British hospitals with white patients," she says. Enslaved Africans on ships were entirely unprotected by the laws safeguarding white patients on land, and had no recourse but to endure unspeakably harsh treatment.

The slave trade may be seen as a starting point for the gross medical inequity in treatment of patients that carried into the late 19th century and beyond—a legacy of disgrace that persisted through the Jim Crow era, was codified in hospital segregation in the 1960s, and shows itself in health disparities between Black and white populations today. Uniquely heinous, the Tuskegee Experiment, in which the U.S. Public Health Service and the Tuskegee Institute in Alabama researched the effects of syphilis in Black men for forty years starting in 1932, represented an utter disregard for these men's humanity. The goal of the study was to learn about the natural course of the disease in men who already had it, and while the researchers didn't *give* participants syphilis at any point during the study (as is sometimes claimed), they did withhold treatment even after it became widely available in the early 1940s and for *nearly three decades* thereafter, causing many men to suffer and die. The researchers never told subjects what the study would entail or got their consent to participate. Treatment was withheld until the Associated Press broke the story in 1972, igniting public outrage.[11] That horrible incident has understandably left a legacy of medical mistrust among many Black people. After Tuskegee, the federal government issued strict regulations to protect human subjects in all the research that it funds. Participants and their families were awarded a $10 million settlement in 1974, and President Bill Clinton issued a formal apology in 1997. But the damage caused can never be undone. "There's a fundamental brokenness in this relationship between Black people and American medicine, medical institutions, medical caregivers, and the healthcare system," Roberts said in a 2020 talk on race and COVID.[12] "It's always been fraught, it's always been broken, and at times it's been deadly."

### The Role of Trauma

The trauma that many marginalized groups have experienced, both at the hands of the medical system and as a result of larger sociocultural forces, surely contributes to reduced well-being.

There is substantial evidence that discrimination and other forms of trauma (including sexual assault, child abuse, being involved in an accident, witnessing someone being injured or killed, or being physically attacked) are linked to health conditions like digestive problems, diabetes, heart disease, and chronic pain—and yet both conventional medicine and wellness culture largely fail to understand or account for trauma. The impact of trauma is also disproportionate, affecting primarily women—who are more than twice as likely as men to have PTSD[13]—and marginalized groups, such as people of color and LGBTQ+ people. "All Black Americans have some degree of PTSD," Monnica Williams, a clinical psychologist and expert in race-based stress and trauma, told the *New York Times* in 2020.[14]

What is trauma? According to the *Diagnostic and Statistical Manual of Mental Disorders* (DSM-5), which is published by the American Psychiatric Association and is widely viewed as the bible for diagnosing mental-health conditions in the U.S., trauma is a response to "actual or threatened death, serious injury, or sexual violence."[15] Yet this definition (as with many things in the DSM) is hotly contested, and in recent years there's been growing recognition that this conception of trauma is too limited. Those types of events can undoubtedly be sources of trauma, but as therapist and author Resmaa Menakem explains, trauma isn't *just* the result of specific, painful incidents like accidents, attacks, and the like. "That may be the case sometimes, but trauma can also be the body's response to a long sequence of smaller wounds," he writes in his bestselling book *My Grandmother's Hands: Racialized Trauma and the Pathway to Mending Our Hearts and Bodies.*[16] "It can be a response to anything that it experiences as too much, too soon, or too fast." Living in poverty, for example, can expose people to many of those smaller wounds—death by a thousand cuts—in the form of daily stress and anxiety. The same is true of experiencing racism, weight stigma, or other forms of discrimination. Living through the COVID-19 pandemic is another form of trauma that has affected many people—including those who experienced the virus directly or up close, such as COVID sufferers and healthcare workers.[17] Even simply being exposed to news about the pandemic, such as consuming content about COVID via social media or traditional media outlets, is associated with increased PTSD symptoms.[18]

Defining PTSD can be similarly complex. Typically characterized by long-term stress and fear that endures even when there is no longer any present danger—as well as other symptoms that may include unpredictable emotions, flashbacks, strained relationships, and physical symptoms—PTSD doesn't necessarily come from one discrete event, and it can persist for long periods of time. In fact, as many as one-third of people who develop PTSD end up having a chronic form of the disorder that can last for years,[19] as has been the case for me. And of course, because of the lack of access to mental-health care in many communities, there are untold numbers of people with trauma and PTSD who never receive a diagnosis or treatment. (Even some people who *are* in therapy may not get a PTSD diagnosis; it took me more than a decade of working with different therapists to get my trauma history and PTSD diagnosed as such.)

Whether diagnosed or not, trauma can provoke a host of physical reactions that are both common and understandable — as one manual on trauma-informed care puts it, "traumatic stress reactions are normal reactions to abnormal circumstances."[20] Physical reactions to trauma that tend to show up right away include gastrointestinal distress, sweating or shivering, faintness, muscle tremors or uncontrollable shaking, elevated heart rate and blood pressure, rapid breathing, extreme fatigue or exhaustion, and a heightened startle response. Delayed or longer-term physical reactions can include hypervigilance, sleep disturbances, an increased focus on and distress about bodily aches and pains, appetite and digestive changes, lowered immunity to colds and infections, persistent fatigue, and elevated cortisol (stress hormone) levels. People who've gone through adverse childhood experiences — traumatic events that are often related to social determinants of health, such as witnessing community violence or experiencing food insecurity — have increased risks of everything from injury to sexually transmitted infections to cancer and diabetes.[21] There's also growing evidence linking trauma to chronic diseases including heart disease and autoimmune conditions.[22]

Reading through this list, it's easy to see why people who've experienced a lot of trauma in their lives might be searching for help for these physical ailments — and vulnerable to wellness-culture promises of relief.

It's also tricky to talk about the possible physical manifestations of trauma without potentially pushing on a long and painful legacy of providers dismissing people's—particularly women's—unexplained illnesses as being purely psychological. This history goes back to the concept of "hysteria," a diagnosis that misogynistically blamed a wide range of health concerns a woman might experience—from irritability and depression, to confusion and forgetfulness, to heart palpitations, muscle spasms, headaches, digestive troubles, and insomnia—on the uterus, the ancient Greek word for which is *hystera*. Though the notion that "hysteria" got its name and definition from the ancient Greek physician Hippocrates has been contested by historians, some doctors in Greek antiquity did seem fixated on the uterus, believing that a "wandering womb" was a cause of numerous diseases and symptoms.[23] Over the centuries the explanation of the mechanisms of and treatments for hysteria changed, but the concept remained a staple of Western medicine and was one of the most common medical diagnoses for many years. In the seventeenth century, hysteria gradually started to be attributed to the brain rather than the uterus, yet it was still considered a predominantly female problem.[24] Eventually hysteria became a mental-health diagnosis, and it was used as a catch-all explanation for any unexplained physical symptoms a woman might experience. Sigmund Freud popularized the notion that hysteria was a response to sexual trauma or repressed sexual urges, and codified the cure: psychoanalysis, which was supposed to uncover the hidden reasons underlying this psychosomatic illness. Therapists continued diagnosing women with hysteria well into the twentieth century. The label was removed from the *Diagnostic and Statistical Manual of Mental Disorders* (DSM) in 1980.

Though it's no longer an official diagnosis, the legacy of hysteria lives on: some doctors tend to treat female patients as if their physical symptoms have exclusively psychological, rather than medical, causes. Any woman who's struggled with a physical ailment that wasn't easily diagnosable has probably encountered at least one provider who made them feel like they were being "hysterical." That's certainly been the case in my and many of my clients' experience. Journalist Meghan O'Rourke wrote that of the nearly one hundred women she interviewed for her book *The Invisible Kingdom* who were eventually diagnosed with autoimmune diseases or other chronic illnesses, "more than 90 percent had been encouraged to seek treatment for anxiety or depression by doctors who told them nothing physical was wrong with them."[25]

Yet the truth is that when it comes to trauma, it's not so easy to untangle the physical from the psychological. Scientists are coming to understand what survivors have long known at an embodied level: that trauma can have real, lasting physical impacts that don't simply go away when the trauma is acknowledged, and that also might not show up on imaging or blood tests. What's more, some people with trauma backgrounds indeed *may* initially present only with physical concerns and may be unaware of the connection between their trauma and the symptoms they're experiencing. Unfortunately, their care providers—whether Western medical doctors or alternative-medicine practitioners—may be equally unaware, resulting in misdiagnoses, frustratingly fruitless bouts of testing and treatment, and ultimately the message from the provider that the issues are "all in your head." But that's a mistaken view of how trauma impacts well-being. Again: while traumatic experiences can cause both physical and psychological reactions, the physical symptoms are real and don't magically disappear once the connection becomes clear to the patient. Nor do they vanish once the trauma is addressed and healed through therapy.

Researchers are still learning how exactly trauma might lead to physical reactions and longer-term outcomes. The answer may lie in trauma's effect on the immune system. The part of our brain responsible for dealing with threats in the environment is called the hypothalamic-pituitary adrenal (HPA) axis, which also plays an important role in the immune response.[26] Chronic stress, especially early in life, can result in HPA dysregulation. Cortisol produced by the HPA basically acts as an on-off switch for the immune system's inflammatory response. (Although inflammation gets a bad rap in wellness culture, it's actually essential for immunity; without inflammation we wouldn't be able to recover from wounds or acute illnesses, and having high levels of inflammation is typical when you're healing from an infection or injury.) If the developing neuroendocrine system is chronically activated, it can lead to too much cortisol in the body, which in turn suppresses the inflammatory response and increases the chance of infection. HPA dysregulation can also result in too *little* cortisol being produced, which can cause the inflammatory response to persist even after it's no longer needed to fight infection. In these ways, childhood trauma in particular can shape the immune system, which can have a significant impact on later-in-life health outcomes including mental and physical health problems, substance abuse, and early mortality.[27] Chronic maternal prenatal stress and anxiety have also been found to be associated with more illnesses and health complaints in newborns.

It might be tempting to think, as wellness culture advocates, that people with trauma-related HPA dysregulation need to go on an "anti-inflammatory" diet, but it's important to remember that food and exercise play a relatively limited role in overall health outcomes—only 10 percent of population health is attributed to them, as we discussed. Anti-inflammatory diets can also trigger seriously disordered eating and a resulting *increase* in chronic stress. Instead, survivors of trauma need accessible and affordable mental-health care, using a trauma-informed care model that helps them feel safe, heard, and empowered in their own care, and avoids retraumatizing them.[28]

As a society, we also need to address the social determinants of health that can lead to trauma in the first place. Rather than focusing on behavioral interventions like diet and exercise, which do nothing to prevent trauma, we need policies to help ensure that people aren't exposed to violence, poverty, discrimination, and other traumatic circumstances.

The mental-health interventions that can help people work through trauma are generally found in the realm of psychotherapy and social work, not alternative medicine. As tempting as it is to believe that simply eating the "right" combination of foods and/or following the "correct" supplement regime (or engaging in self-care, like baths or a meditation app) can reverse the effects of trauma, the reality is that recovery is much harder, slower work. Trauma can take years, even decades, to untangle. "Trauma is all about speed and reflexivity—which is why, in addressing trauma, each of us needs to work through it slowly, over time," writes Menakem. Getting support is key, but access to mental-health care is often limited, especially for the most marginalized. Somatic work—reconnecting to the body—is also important (indeed, many trauma specialists say essential) for recovery, which is why trauma therapy often includes work on noticing and experiencing physical sensations. This is also where practices like yoga, meditation, breathwork, and other mind-body modalities can come into play as adjunctive therapies. Trauma is an embodied experience, creating physical responses that are often deeply embedded in the body, so trauma healing must be embodied as well.

Just as in other areas of wellness culture, though, practices meant to heal trauma can easily be co-opted or abused. Julian Walker experienced this firsthand. Walker, a yoga teacher, writer, and cohost of the *Conspirituality* podcast (as well as a coauthor of the forthcoming book *Conspirituality: How New Age Conspiracy Theories Became a Health Threat*), has been in the yoga and wellness space for nearly thirty years, and has been skeptical of many practices endorsed by that community for just as long. Still, he says, even though he'd long believed that "approaches to personal growth should be grounded in reality and should not be another way of psychologically fooling ourselves, or of enacting spiritual bypass," he ended up being drawn into a group that he now recognizes had a bit of a cultlike mentality—especially around trauma and what it takes to heal from it.

He was in his early twenties when he started taking classes from a well-known yoga teacher and alternative healer, who soon became his employer and mentor. Though he thinks that her efforts were well intentioned, he says she seemed to believe that she somehow drew people to her who had painful repressed memories, and that she alone could help them recall them and ultimately heal from their trauma (despite having no formal training in psychotherapy). "It was appealing to me because there was more of a psychological component," says Walker. "It was about getting real. It was about facing your darkness in a way that a lot of the rest of the yoga community and the New Age world was in denial of."

Taking stock of oneself in that way can be valuable when done with the right support, but Walker now sees that the approach of this particular community was anything but responsible. The yoga teacher influenced Walker to believe that he must have suffered abuse in his family—specifically at the hands of his father—that he had buried so deeply he now couldn't remember it.

The notion that it's common to have absolutely no memory of physical or sexual abuse endured as a child is highly controversial and has been largely discredited since the 1990s, when it flourished in certain circles. At the time, some psychotherapists viewed symptoms of anxiety, mood, personality, or eating disorders as signs that patients were repressing memories of abuse.[29] Techniques like hypnosis, guided imagery, dream interpretation, and other methods were used, ostensibly to bring repressed memories into consciousness, often with a strong element of suggestion from the therapist. The "satanic panic" that swept the U.S. in the late 1980s and '90s was driven in large part by therapists supposedly uncovering repressed memories of presumed ritual abuse in their patients.

Research eventually showed that suggestive interviewing techniques could actually implant false autobiographical memories. The concept of repressed memories has been found to run contrary to substantial evidence demonstrating that people generally remember the central features of traumatic events (even if they're fuzzy on the smaller details), and that having zero memory of such events is rare.[30] Indeed, people with PTSD often experience flashbacks and intrusive memories of traumatic incidents—the opposite of memory repression. In the more than twelve thousand documented allegations of sexual abuse by satanic cults through late 1994, investigators weren't able to substantiate a single one.[31] A large body of research published in psychological, psychiatric, and legal journals concluded that the notion of repressed memories is at best filled with holes—and at worst, particularly when used in court, defamatory and libelous, with false "repressed" memories resulting in unjust convictions.[32]

Yet belief in repressed memories—and modern-day versions of the satanic panic—live on today in wellness and self-development spaces. One of its most popular proponents is Teal Swan, a spiritual influencer whose controversial tactics involve encouraging her followers—many of whom are struggling with depression and suicidal ideation—to visualize dying, which mental-health professionals have pointed out is extremely dangerous. Swan has no mental-health credentials, and she's made many outlandish claims, including saying that she's an alien from another planet and that she can X-ray people with her mind. But perhaps her most sensational claim is that she endured horrific, satanic ritual abuse as a child—memories of which she repressed but later uncovered through therapy. Her therapist was Barbara Snow, a well-known proponent of the problematic theory of repressed memories and a central figure in the satanic panic of the 1980s and '90s.[33] And now Swan has taken on Snow's mantle, spreading the dubious idea of repressed memories to hundreds of thousands of people through her popular YouTube channel and social media pages.

Walker, for his part, came to realize that his belief that he'd been abused by his father and repressed the memory simply wasn't true. When he was in the grip of the idea, the pressure from his yoga community to believe it was very powerful. "There was a certain amount of approval and recognition that you were moving forward on the path when you started to uncover what those repressed memories were," he says. And the need for that approval was powerful for him because although he didn't actually endure child abuse, he did have trauma in his past that made him crave the sense of identity and community—and the intense relationship with a charismatic teacher—that the group was offering.

He had spent a difficult and painful couple of years searching for repressed memories, which deeply damaged his relationships with his family; though he has since reconciled with his parents, he says his relationship with his younger brother has never been the same. Eventually he got help from a psychotherapist, let go of the notion of repressed memories, and moved into a deeper and more nuanced understanding of his own past. That process allowed him to see that his yoga teacher and mentor was so caught up in her own beliefs about the nature of trauma that she couldn't help but foist them onto others. Now, he views her approach as "a very black-and-white or oversimplified idea of how people heal from whatever their early life experiences are," he says.

Unfortunately, wellness culture is rife with black-and-white views on mental health that fly in the face of what we know about trauma and social determinants.

## The Pitfalls of Manifesting

In the corner of the wellness world devoted to mental health, there's a particularly pernicious idea that goes something like this: all the mental illnesses in the *DSM,* as well as any other mental-health condition people might experience, have one common root, which is a "victim mentality" or "victim consciousness." Seeing your suffering as having any external cause at all—whether it's poverty, lack of access to healthcare, discrimination, abuse, or the virus that causes COVID-19—is victim consciousness. And the solution, according to this worldview, is to *think* your way into a different state (as well as sometimes to change your diet and take supplements, which we'll get to shortly). This idea of changing your mindset to change your life is not meant in the sense of traditional psychotherapy, where you might try to change your habitual thoughts and reactions to better cope with a bad situation, or treat yourself with compassion while going through it, or even focus on your strengths and how they can help you overcome obstacles. Instead, the common wellness-culture view of mental health says that you *literally* create reality with your mind, like magic.

This is the "law of attraction"—the idea that your thoughts "attract" things into your life in a very concrete way. There's a lot of pseudoscientific talk of "frequencies" and "vibrations": high-frequency or "high-vibe" thoughts supposedly attract good things, whereas "low-vibe" thoughts—that pesky victim consciousness—attract the opposite. For anyone struggling with difficult life circumstances, this all can feel incredibly shaming and blaming—but then that's just framed as more victim mentality, to be eradicated by raising your frequency.

Few would dispute the fact that getting locked into an identity solely as a victim is disempowering, detracting from your agency and ability to cope. And some people have indeed found solace in ideas and practices related to the law of attraction, like affirmations and vision boards (typically in conjunction with other forms of psychological support). But the full-blown idea—that you literally create your reality with your thoughts—is harmful to well-being in many ways, creating anxiety and self-blame and dissuading people from getting the help they need to care for their mental health.

The 2006 film and bestselling book *The Secret* helped entrench the law of attraction in wellness culture, popularizing the practice of "manifesting"—thinking your way to positive outcomes. "What you think about, you bring about," *The Secret* proclaims. "Your whole life is a manifestation of the thoughts that go on in your head."[34] Of course there's truth to the idea that your thoughts affect your emotions and behaviors and therefore can affect the direction of your life. But the law of attraction stretches this truth beyond the limits of reality and into the realm of magical thinking. It says that "your thoughts become things"—tangible things, like money and parking spots and bad haircuts. Your thoughts are a magician's wand, making objects appear and disappear. Got sick, lost your job, or went through a breakup? *The Secret* argues that you manifested it, because everything in your life—good, bad, or otherwise—is *literally* a product of your thoughts.

The law of attraction dates back at least to the New Thought movement of the 1800s, a key forerunner of much of the New Age thinking that underlies today's wellness culture. New Thought was popularized by Phineas Parkhurst Quimby, a hypnotist who had suffered from tuberculosis as a child and believed he had cured himself through exposure to fresh air.[35] From this experience and his studies in hypnosis (or "mesmerism," as it was known at the time), he developed the conviction that all illness is essentially a matter of the mind—caused by mistaken beliefs—and that the cure is simply correcting those beliefs. Considered a cult by some scholars, New Thought had many intellectual descendants, from eclectic spiritual belief systems like the New Age movement to overtly religious philosophies including Christian Science and the Prosperity Gospel. Decades before *The Secret*, two other wildly popular self-help books that came out of New Thought were *Think and Grow Rich* (1937), by Napoleon Hill (who was later found to have scammed numerous business associates and invented large chunks of his books) and *The Power of Positive Thinking* (1952), by pastor Norman Vincent Peale (an ardent Hill fan whom Donald Trump cites as his major religious influence).[36] Both books are problematic in many ways, but they've had an enduring influence for their simple advice that by changing your mindset you can change your life.

Again, there's some truth to that idea; changing how you think about and relate to your circumstances can have an impact on well-being, and it's at the core of evidence-based therapy methods like cognitive-behavioral therapy. But in the law of attraction, that grain of truth gets distorted into the false belief that positive thinking is the one and only secret to a good life, and that your thoughts determine everything that comes your way.

The law of attraction has had a huge impact on wellness culture over the years. It's been embraced by many of the biggest names in wellness and self-care, including Deepak Chopra and Oprah Winfrey. It's become a hashtag with millions of posts on social media, a sea of quotes about vibrations and the universe and mind healing. And it drew an even larger audience during the COVID-19 pandemic. Between March and July of 2020, Google searches for the term "manifesting" jumped more than 550 percent.[37] Teenagers on TikTok started sharing their own version of the practice, called scripting—repeatedly writing down a wish in order to make it come true. "Shut up I'm manifesting" became, in the words of one reporter, "among the defining memes of 2020."[38]

It's understandable that the law of attraction would become increasingly popular during the early days of the pandemic, when everything felt so out of our control; in times of over-whelming uncertainty, the idea that we can simply think our way into a better reality is hugely appealing. Yet although that kind of magical thinking might feel comforting, it also can be detrimental.

For one thing, it ignores the very real fact that social deter-minants play a major role in life and health outcomes. As another meme that made the rounds a few years ago put it, "maybe you manifested it, maybe it's white privilege." Consider this passage from *The Secret* about how the law of attraction sup-posedly applies to money: "People who have drawn wealth into their lives used The Secret, whether consciously or uncon-sciously. They think thoughts of abundance and wealth, and they do not allow any contradictory thoughts to take root in their minds. Their predominant thoughts are of wealth. They only *know* wealth, and nothing else exists in their minds."[39] It's easy to "only *know* wealth" when you're already living it—and perhaps even when you're fairly close to it, and not facing struc-tural barriers that prevent you from getting the rest of the way there. But if your everyday experience is grinding poverty and obstacles to advancement, where you're constantly having to put off one bill to pay another, how exactly is it possible to have "nothing else exist in your mind" other than thoughts of wealth? You'd have to be completely divorced from reality.

Another problem with this lionization of positive thinking is that it cuts people off from feeling the full range of human emo-tions. When "low-vibe" thoughts are seen as the source of all your troubles, it's hard not to become terrified of having even the most minor complaint. Nitika Chopra, (no relation to Deepak), the founder of the chronic-illness community Chroni-con learned that lesson firsthand from her foray into the self-improvement world in her early twenties. "I didn't want to feel even one 'negative' thought because all the self-help and well-ness gurus kept telling me that if you aren't thinking positive thoughts you are making yourself sick, poor, and unlovable," she wrote in a 2021 newsletter.[40]

In my research for this book, I felt something similar. I'd never read *The Secret* (though I had encountered a couple of the other self-help books published later that incorporated some of its ideas without naming them), but when I finally flipped through it, my anxiety spiked. I began to police my thoughts in a way that I hadn't done since my early twenties—when I thankfully found a psychotherapist who focused on self-compassion and radical acceptance, and learned to stop being so hard on myself. For hours after skimming *The Secret*, I felt an irrational fear bubbling up: that thinking the "wrong" thing would cause me to lose all the well-being and life stability I've managed to eke out (through a combination of hard work, good luck, and systemic advantages, not manifesting).

It turns out that this is a common and understandable response to being exposed to the law of attraction, especially for people who have preexisting mental-health conditions. The experience is not unlike what psychologists call "thought-action fusion"—the belief that your thoughts can cause actions (if you think about getting into a car accident, you will) and/or that thoughts are morally equivalent to actions (if you think about hitting your partner, it's just as bad as if you'd actually done it).[41] Thought-action fusion is a common feature in obsessive-compulsive disorder, anxiety disorders, eating disorders, and depression, which makes manifesting risky for people with these conditions. "In the therapy sessions that I attend each week for anxiety and obsessive compulsive disorder, I spend a lot of time learning the opposite lesson: that thoughts do not equal reality," journalist Shayla Love wrote for *Vice* in a piece about the harms of the law of attraction.[42] "*These are just thoughts*, my therapist has taught me to say...I can observe them and let them be, and not worry that they'll leak out through my ears and somehow infiltrate my everyday life."

My own therapy for anxiety and PTSD has focused on similar concepts: feelings aren't facts (though they can have valuable things to teach us). I can't predict the future (even if a current situation reminds me of one from my past). And just because I'm worried about something—or, conversely, just because I really want something—doesn't mean it's going to happen. Internalizing these ideas over the course of many years has had a profoundly positive impact on my life, allowing me to have better relationships and reach more long-term goals than I could ever have imagined—and the law of attraction threatens to undermine those hard-won understandings. It's no wonder even a quick perusal of *The Secret* would stir up some anxiety.

Manifesting isn't only dangerous for people with preexisting mental-health conditions, though. As cognitive neuroscientist Rhiannon Jones told Love for that article, the practice of manifesting might be enough to trigger anxiety and obsessive thoughts even in people who never had those symptoms before.

That might help explain why, in this age of rampant wellness culture, getting a physical-health diagnosis—or even just having physical symptoms—can (for some people) quickly lead to anxiety and obsession. One of the long-standing corollaries of the law of attraction is that illness is caused by negative thoughts, and that if you're sick it's simply because you need to raise your vibration. For example, popular self-help author (and not-as-popular 2020 Democratic presidential candidate) Marianne Williamson wrote in her 1992 book *A Return to Love*, "sickness is an illusion and does not exist," and "cancer and AIDS and other physical illnesses are physical manifestations of a psychic scream."[43] During the 2020 campaign, many disability-rights activists wrote with alarm about Williamson's ableist rhetoric, which included this now-deleted tweet: "spirit self, which is the true Self, cannot be disabled." Williamson has since apologized for many of those statements, and she's denied she ever said that negative thinking causes people to get sick. But some other high-profile wellness influencers have said as much—and gone even further. One of them is Kelly Brogan.

A former *goop* contributor, Brogan calls herself a "holistic psychiatrist," though in 2020 she did not renew her board certification in psychiatry.[44] As of this writing she still advertises herself as an MD, but she's become notorious for her dangerous and ableist views, including arguing that no one ever needs to be on psychiatric medication and implying that taking meds makes people weak. Her work revolves around getting her followers to ditch their medications and convert to her "lifestyle medicine" program, which involves some standard wellness-culture fare (such as a particular style of yoga, supplements, and of course a gluten-free, "ancestral" diet that demonizes "industrial foods") as well as some more extreme and dangerous practices including coffee enemas.

Her extreme views go even further, though. She also argues that no one needs to use conventional medicine for any reason, including to treat cancer and acute infections. She's stridently anti-vaccine. She claims that instead of using Western medicine, people need to think their way out of their symptoms—she's a vocal proponent of the idea that "victim consciousness" creates illness. She's written admiringly about a fringe German medical philosophy that argues "the body develops cancer as a part of a highly meaningful biological program that limits itself once the original psychic conflict is resolved...this process [that causes cancer] spontaneously resolves (with the help of the inner microbiome) when the conflict is addressed."[45] The founder of that sect, an anti-Semitic German doctor who at the age of fifty was stripped of his medical license following the death "under inhumane circumstances" of patients in his care, promoted the baseless and vile conspiracy theory that chemotherapy was invented by Jewish doctors as a means of exterminating non-Jews (which is also nonsensical, since chemotherapy has actually saved countless lives). He died in 2017 in Norway, having continued to "treat" patients in more than five different countries for at least twenty-one years after the revocation of his license, and having been run out of France and Spain.[46]

Brogan not only claims that so-called victim consciousness can cause illness, but she also denies that other causes even exist—including germs. She's become one of a number of wellness influencers who, without any good evidence, have started to dispute that microbes are responsible for infectious diseases. She has derided the well-established science by boiling it down to "little invisible pathogens, you know, that randomly jump around from person to person."[47] She has argued that the COVID-19 pandemic is not real, that the virus that causes COVID may not exist, and that deaths from the virus are instead likely caused by fear.[48]

This view—and more generally, the notion that sickness is a manifestation of low-vibe thoughts—exemplifies the "it's all in your head" rhetoric that has plagued women's health for centuries. Brogan and other wellness influencers with similar views sometimes invoke feminism, pointing out that Western medicine has ignored and harmed women in many ways. And indeed this is true, but these influencers mix this grain of truth into a stew of wild, baseless arguments—like Brogan's assertion in a now-deleted blog post that antibiotics are "the emblematic sacrament of the patriarchy."[49] Proponents of this view might think they're somehow helping women, but in denying the reality of diseases like COVID and blaming them entirely on emotions, they're engaging in the same kind of gaslighting they accuse conventional medicine of doing. They're re-creating the provider-patient dynamic that existed in the days of "hysteria" diagnoses, but now under the guise of feminism—which makes it all the more confusing for people in their audiences to untangle.

And those audiences are massive, thanks to an online environment that privileges mis- and disinformation, as we'll discuss next.

# CHAPTER 4

# Mis- and Disinformation

When I first started struggling with a constellation of symptoms that doctors couldn't explain, it was a simpler time to seek out information. The year was 2003, and the only social media site I was on at the time (or even had heard of) was Friendster, one of the original social networks and the progenitor of the friend-request system that Facebook later popularized. Unlike the Facebook of today, Friendster didn't have creepy ads that tracked you across the Internet. I can't even remember if it had ads at all back then (though by 2004 it did, according to a *Wall Street Journal* article from that year with the now quaint headline "Advertisers Seek Friends on Social-Networking Sites"[1]).

I didn't post about my health concerns on Friendster, though. Instead, I got my health information by googling around, finding and peeking into message boards dedicated to particular diseases—celiac disease, thyroiditis, digestive disorders. I never posted myself, but I lurked and picked up some ideas from those forums, such as the notion that gluten might be at the root of my disparate symptoms (which I much later learned definitely was not the case), or the idea that something hormonal might be going on beyond my thyroid problem.

Yet much of the content in those spaces never really resonated with me—perhaps because in some cases (as with the celiac board) I never actually had the disease, or maybe because, though I was desperate for answers, the people on those boards seemed so much more desperate and willing to try extreme things. Though I engaged in many disordered eating behaviors and was obsessed with "healthy" diets and cutting out certain foods, the severe and esoteric restrictions and unproven wellness-culture practices that some of the people on those message boards were advocating didn't feel right to me at first glance, and it was fairly easy to forget about them and move on.

If I were going through the same thing as a young person today, I have no doubt my experience would be very different.

Now, arcane and often bizarre food restrictions are peddled by wellness influencers with millions of followers, and even casually viewing or "liking" those pages can cause sophisticated algorithms to serve up increasingly extreme diets and harmful practices. Those same algorithms can drive wellness-seekers to dangerous pseudoscience and misinformation. Dubious alternative-medicine advice that was still very much on the fringes back when I was first struggling with chronic illness now often shows up on the first page of search results, driven by personalization algorithms and those sites' well-honed social media and search-engine-optimization strategies.

Much of this shift is a result of the modern attention economy, and what author and social psychologist Shoshana Zuboff calls "surveillance capitalism"—the collection and sale of our personal data (search histories, social media likes, page views, age, location, etc.) to advertisers, who use it to precisely target us with ads designed to capture our attention far better than non-personalized ads ever could. The technology of surveillance capitalism is what allows those creepy ads to follow us around the Internet, but its influence is far more insidious than just making you buy some skin serum you might otherwise have forgotten about. This technology also makes people vulnerable to mis- and disinformation, opening us up to scams and conspiracy theories—and ultimately compromising both our individual health and our collective well-being.

## Misinformation and the Attention Economy

Healthcare professionals and consumers alike have been concerned about the quality of health information on the Internet since the early days of what was then known as the World Wide Web. In the mid-1990s, doctors and information specialists began to sound the alarm about the dangers of having a space where anyone could say whatever they wanted about health-related topics, without any of the usual editing and filtering out of misinformation that happens in traditional publishing.[2] Initially, this growing concern over the quality of online health content led the medical community to push for greater regulation, but it quickly became clear that content was proliferating too quickly for regulation to have any hope of keeping up.

Instead, doctors and other medical professionals began advocating for market-based strategies to prevent the emergence of misinformation and combat what did get through. A number of academic and commercial sources launched accreditation initiatives, creating criteria for judging the quality of health information that appeared on various websites.[3] These initiatives included things like "seals of approval" and "awards" placed prominently on health sites, which at the time may have felt slightly less futile than that sounds today.

Eventually, these initiatives attracted the attention of the World Health Organization (WHO), which wanted to launch one of its own. The WHO got in touch with the organization that essentially runs the Internet—the Internet Corporation for Assigned Names and Numbers, or ICANN—and submitted a proposal to create a top-level ".health" domain that would signify a website met stringent quality and ethical criteria. Health websites wouldn't *have* to use the .health domain, but it would act as a reliable filter for users who wanted to search only credible sources.

ICANN's chairman at the time said it seemed like a beneficial tool and encouraged the WHO to pursue the idea further, but his support was no match for the opposition. In late 2000, numerous stakeholders successfully argued that the Internet couldn't be regulated in this way, that users were already savvy enough to recognize online charlatans, and that no one organization should have the power to pass judgment on thousands upon thousands of websites.[4] Even then, not long after the advent of social media in its nascent form, there was a reflexive resistance to the possibility of having health-related mis- and disinformation automatically flagged. Opponents of regulation framed their objections in the broadest possible terms — it was, they said, a matter of nothing less than individual liberty. In ascendancy was a free-market neoliberal belief that would go on to change the face of healthcare: the idea that care is not a right but an individual responsibility. As such, the thinking went, people were free to educate themselves (or not) about health-related matters. In this view, regulating what people could say about health would amount to restriction of free speech.

Flash forward thirty years, and we're having a not dissimilar debate — about whether social media companies have the right, and a responsibility, to remove health mis- and disinformation from their platforms.

In my view it's more urgent than ever that tech companies step in and stop the spread of false health and wellness claims online, but at this point they have no real incentive to do that. Under Section 230 of the Communications Decency Act, tech companies aren't legally liable for user-generated content, which means people can say whatever they want on social media and other tech platforms without those platforms having to worry about being sued when users inevitably post false, libelous, or otherwise harmful things.[5] Traditional publishers don't have the same freedoms and are often rightly held liable for the content they create and disseminate. But under Section 230, platforms like Facebook, Twitter, YouTube, and others aren't considered "publishers."

That wasn't always the case. In 1995, the brokerage firm Stratton Oakmont (whose cofounder Jordan Belfort was portrayed by Leonardo DiCaprio in *The Wolf of Wall Street*) brought a successful defamation suit against the Internet service provider Prodigy, which the New York Supreme Court deemed to be a publisher. The rationale was that Prodigy had exerted editorial oversight by moderating some posts and prohibiting certain content, and therefore it wasn't simply acting as a content distributor, in the manner of a newsstand or bookstore. This decision riled two members of Congress, who worried that it would make tech companies less likely to moderate *any* content, leading every website to become overrun with pornography. So they worked together to get a pivotal sentence included in the 1996 Communications Decency Act: "No provider or user of an interactive computer service shall be treated as the publisher or speaker of any information provided by another information content provider."[6]

Section 230 is the foundation of online life today—"the 26 words that created the Internet," as it's come to be known. Social media probably never would have become this big, this wild, this unwieldy (if it existed at all) without Section 230. Amending it to close the "publisher" loophole, at least in certain cases—which lawmakers have floated several times over the years, with varying levels of bipartisan support—would force social media companies to ensure that their platforms don't allow mis- and disinformation to go viral. The move would dramatically curtail the spread of false information. So far, as of this writing, that hasn't happened.

A key reason tech companies are slow to act in preventing false claims is financial. Social media algorithms are designed to promote engagement and keep people liking, clicking, and sharing on the platforms, which in turn brings in more advertising revenue for them. And what kind of content does that best? Content that provokes anger and disgust, uses moral-emotional language, and/or introduces seemingly novel information, as numerous studies have found.[7] That's why the YouTube algorithm tends to pick up and promote videos that have words like "hates," "destroys," "obliterates," and "slams" in the title, and why every word of moral outrage added to a tweet raises the retweet rate by an average of 20 percent. As journalist Johann Hari wrote in his 2022 book *Stolen Focus*, "if it's more enraging, it's more engaging."[8]

Falsehoods often hit all of those notes—novelty, disgust, and moral outrage—and that combination can make them spread like wildfire. In a 2018 study, a group of researchers tracked more than 125,000 rumors disseminated by more than three million Twitter users, and found that false claims diffused significantly further, faster, and more broadly than the truth.[9] The truth rarely reached more than a thousand people, while viral misinformation routinely racked up audiences of between one thousand and one hundred thousand—and it spread about six times more quickly. False information was also 70 percent more likely to be retweeted than the truth, and it was mostly real people—not bots—doing the retweeting. The people spreading misinformation, in turn, are rewarded with likes and shares, which reinforces this dynamic. In the current social media landscape, lies often go viral while the truth languishes.

That's true for rumors about all kinds of subjects, from politics to celebrity gossip, but false information about health and wellness is particularly prolific. As one physician and TikTok influencer estimated in 2022, "For every large creator [on the platform] who is genuinely evidence-based, you've got 50 or 60 big creators who spread misinformation" about health.[10] That includes harmful diet advice, unsubstantiated claims that food ingredients cause cancer, the false notion that only "natural" medicine can be trusted, myths about contraception, recipes for potentially deadly "herbal abortions," and many, many more untrue and misleading ideas, across all social media platforms and related technologies such as YouTube.

And when misinformation deals with health and wellness, it poses an extreme risk to anyone in its path. Perhaps the deadliest kind of all is vaccine misinformation, which we'll discuss in detail in the next chapter. A nationally representative survey of nearly twenty-five hundred U.S. adults by researchers at the University of Pennsylvania in the spring and fall of 2019 (when the U.S. experienced its largest measles outbreak in more than 25 years) found that up to 20 percent of respondents were at least somewhat misinformed about vaccines—and that people tended to become more misinformed with greater social media use.[11] Respondents who reported increased exposure to content about the measles, mumps, and rubella (MMR) vaccine on social media were more likely to become more misinformed about vaccines over time, whereas those who reported increased exposure to news from traditional media outlets tended to become *less* misinformed (that is, better informed) about vaccines. This study wasn't a randomized controlled trial, so it's possible that other factors could explain the link, but the timing is suggestive—becoming more misinformed came *after* exposure to social media, not before.

Other research conducted during the COVID-19 pandemic has linked greater exposure to vaccine misinformation to a lower likelihood of getting vaccinated. For example, a representative survey of six hundred adults in the state of Florida in 2021 found that among people who didn't report any exposure to misinformation about COVID-19 vaccines, roughly 74 percent of respondents were vaccinated.[12] That number fell to just 63 percent among people who'd been exposed to one misinformation theme, and 52 percent for those who'd been exposed to six or more. Crucially, the link between exposure to misinformation and vaccination held true even when controlling for other demographics that might account for the difference in vaccination status, such as age, race, and political affiliation.

A series of randomized controlled trials from 2018 with more than eighteen hundred total participants found that even a single exposure to a piece of misinformation can make people more likely to judge it as accurate in the future, provided it's not wildly implausible (such as a statement like "the Earth is a perfect square").[13] This "illusory truth effect" held even when fake-news stories were labeled as disputed by fact-checkers—which has often been the solution of social media companies to the problem of misinformation on their platforms. Given that social media is a fount of falsehoods about wellness, spending time on social platforms is likely to increase people's exposure to wellness mis- and disinformation that, in turn, comes to seem more plausible over time.

Traditional media also bear some responsibility for the proliferation of health and wellness misinformation. Numerous studies have found that legacy media and news organizations around the world have allowed the COVID-19 "infodemic" to spread relatively unchecked.[14] Of course not all media outlets are equally culpable. A 2022 study found that starting in May 2021, watching Fox News directly caused higher levels of vaccine hesitancy and lower levels of vaccine uptake than watching other cable outlets; viewing MSNBC and CNN had no effect on either.[15] The researchers found that, even controlling for partisan affiliation and political ideology, the effect of watching Fox News on vaccine uptake remained, and that it was likely the network's uniquely vaccine-skeptical narrative that drove many viewers to eschew the vaccine. Another study from 2022 found that college students who were more conservative were more likely to consume news from right-wing outlets, which in turn was linked to increases in vaccine hesitancy.[16] Although other outlets also reported some misinformation, particularly early in the pandemic (largely a function of the fact that no one really knew much about the virus in those early days), misinformation has continued to proliferate in right-wing outlets. QAnon (the baseless and bizarre conspiracy theory that says prominent Democrats and Hollywood stars are part of a satanic global cabal that kills babies and drinks their blood in order to stay young), vaccine misinformation, and bogus COVID cures all have been promoted by right-wing media.[17]

Some of this misinformation is actually better referred to as *disinformation*, or falsehoods knowingly spread with the intent to deceive or mislead. Granted, in many cases it's hard to ever truly know another person's intentions, but sometimes circumstances make it clear where people stand. For example, a lawyer for Alex Jones—the right-wing media host who promotes false health and wellness claims, anti-vax rhetoric, and supplements along-side political conspiracy theories—argued in a child-custody case that in his public rants Jones is "playing a character; he is a performance artist."[18] Jones's former cameraman Josh Owens says the whole organization was in on the act: "I was part of that machine, we lied, and it was intentional," Owens told WNYC's *On the Media* in 2022.[19] Similarly, when Fox News airs anti-vaccine content nearly every day while simultaneously mandating that employees get vaccinated, it's hard to argue that the network isn't intentionally misleading its viewers.[20]

In a more indirect way, some social media companies might be said to be purveyors of disinformation because they knew their products were spreading harmful falsehoods and chose to let it continue. As Facebook whistleblower Frances Haugen revealed in 2021, the company's own internal research showed that its algorithms were pushing teenage girls who expressed an interest in dieting or "healthy eating" toward increasingly extreme weight-loss and pro-anorexia content.[21] Because the algorithms are weighted to favor novel and controversial information, extreme and unsubstantiated diet claims get amplified more than benign and commonplace posts about nutrition. This was a serious problem with the algorithm that Facebook confirmed in its own testing, Haugen said, and yet it did nothing about it for years. "We make body image issues worse for one in three teen girls," said one slide from a 2019 Facebook internal presentation. "Thirty-two percent of teen girls said that when they felt bad about their bodies, Instagram made them feel worse," another presentation from March 2020 said. "Teens told us that they don't like the amount of time they spend on the app but feel like they have to be present," an Instagram research manager told colleagues. "They often feel 'addicted' and know that what they're seeing is bad for their mental health but feel unable to stop themselves."

According to the internal documents that Haugen made public (now known as the Facebook Papers), top Facebook executives have seen this research, which was cited in a 2020 presentation given to Mark Zuckerberg. The company's knowledge of these issues likely goes back even further: James P. Steyer, the CEO and founder of the children's media and advocacy organization Common Sense Media, testified before Congress in December 2021 that ten years prior, he wrote a book about Facebook that contained information about teen body-image issues linked to use of the platform. At that time, he said, the heads of Facebook—whom he met with repeatedly—knew their product was negatively influencing young people's body image and chose not to act.[22]

The real-world consequences of mis- and disinformation can be particularly severe for communities of color. Take the false and discriminatory "Chinese virus" narrative about COVID-19. Months before the virus reached pandemic status and Donald Trump was regularly repeating anti-Asian racist rhetoric, Australian newspapers ran some particularly bad headlines, like *The Herald Sun*'s racist pun about the "Chinese Virus Pandamonium" or the *Daily Telegraph*'s "China Kids Stay Home." As early as

January 2020, that narrative was getting amplified on social media and had sparked racist comments and abuse toward Asian people in many parts of the world.[23] The situation only got worse as the pandemic wore on, with reports of physical violence and at least one death—an eighty-four-year-old Thai man named Vicha Ratanapakdee—attributed to anti-Asian racism.[24]

In the U.S., where the majority of social media companies are based, the fundamental belief in personal responsibility puts the burden on individuals to determine what information is credible and who to trust—yet the structure of social media platforms makes it hard to do that. Social media flattens sources of information, so that a person with education, work experience, and credentials in a particular field (such as health/wellness) is presented in very much the same way as an influencer perhaps speaking solely from their own experience—and the influencer might have a similar or greater number of followers, lending them the appearance of greater trustworthiness. Sometimes it's not even an influencer, but just a regular person whose testimonial about a certain wellness practice goes viral. There's certainly nothing wrong with sharing personal experiences; indeed, it's powerful and important in many instances, and it can help others find connections and support that they aren't getting from the healthcare system. But in matters of wellness, it can be dangerous to model your own behavior on a social media personality whose only real evidence is "this worked for me."

Moreover, this flattening of information sources creates a relativism that can easily be exploited by purveyors of mis- and disinformation. Not only does social media often give greater reach to influencers who may not know what they're talking about, but it also places well-conducted scientific research on the same footing as anecdotes and non-peer-reviewed preprint studies, blurring them all together in one endless scroll. In the process, it creates the illusion that all of these sources are equally valid, which may allow false information to gain traction.

It's tempting to think that you can simply be aware of this flattening effect and be discerning about your sources of information, but in fact it's much more difficult than you think to differentiate. Even professional critics of the phenomenon find it tough. "It is so hard to convince myself to ignore things from randos online," said Charlie Warzel, a tech journalist who has been covering social media and the Internet for years, in a 2022 interview for *The Atlantic.*[25] "I remember seeing all these doom posts during 2020 about COVID and realizing they were from just…random anonymous people. And I could rationally tell myself to ignore them, but my brain had a hard time letting go of those signals." In fact our brains are wired to zero in on negative information, a vulnerability that the platforms are designed to exploit. Individual users, no matter how savvy, aren't necessarily equipped to filter out the noise.

Given all these problems, I can't help but wonder how much less of a mess we'd be in now if Section 230 had been implemented differently or not at all, or if there had been some effort at the outset to draw clearer lines between credible health content (including genuine areas of scientific debate and inquiry) and misleading pseudoscience. How many people might have avoided rabbit holes of wellness misinformation created by algorithms that reward controversy over contemplation and sensationalism over sound evidence? How much more quickly could the U.S. have addressed COVID-19? How many lives might have been saved in the process? Of course the Internet isn't to blame for all our cultural ills, many of which predated it by hundreds of years. But online health mis- and disinformation is more harmful and has more far-reaching consequences than may have been imagined at the birth of the Internet.

## *Harm to Collective Well-Being*

You pick up your phone to look for something specific—say it's directions. But before you can even get to the maps app, you notice several notifications on your lock screen. Three new people commented on your latest photo, and you have a couple of new replies to one of your comments. Opening the phone, you see red bubbles on seven different apps, each blaring the number of unread notifications: thirteen new Instagram likes and shares, five retweets and comments, two Facebook messages, eight friend requests—plus four missed calls, nine new text messages, and thirty-six unread emails. You click Facebook Messenger to see who's messaging you, then pop over to Twitter to make sure the new comments are all positive. Next you tap your phone app to confirm that the calls are all spam and nothing urgent, then scan your text messages and reply to a few. Why did you open your phone again? Right, directions. Just need to check the Facebook invite to see where you're going, and while you're at it you might as well accept a couple of those friend requests. As you're doing that, another Twitter notification pops up. Someone just mentioned you . . . don't you want to know what they're saying?

Today's technology is great at commanding our attention through simple prompts like this. Those red balloons tallying our unread messages feel like red marks on a math test totaling up the sum of our errors, our failures. Making them disappear feels like progress, like cleaning up a mess or checking items off a checklist. Being notified that people are writing to you in a public (or semi-public) forum is compelling, because if you're not there to see their comments, it kind of feels like everyone is hanging out without you—or talking about you behind your back. Racking up likes and positive comments can seem like an antidote to those worries, at least for a moment, but the feeling never really lasts. Soon you're back to feeling bored, antsy, uneasy about your worth. You need another hit.

If you feel this way in relationship to your phone, you're not alone—and it's not your fault. Social platforms were designed to exploit basic facts and foibles of human psychology in service of the attention economy. This includes not just the novelty and moral outrage that keep us engaged and clicking, but also the fundamental desires to be loved and to belong—or even just to be seen and recognized. Social media creates a "synthetic version" of the desire for recognition, as news anchor Chris Hayes puts it in a 2021 piece for *The New Yorker*, and that synthetic version isn't fulfilling, because interacting with strangers online lacks the mutuality that's required in a relationship in order for us to feel truly seen.[26] Yet we keep coming back for more, because the platforms have trained us to accept that simulacrum of connection as the real thing. In a sense, social media relationships are like diet food, temporarily taking the edge off the hunger for connection but never really satisfying it.

Granted, social media has fostered real-world connections for many people, myself included. For some marginalized people it's been especially important, allowing them to find each other, organize, document abuses such as police violence against Black people, and get backing for their causes. It's helped people with chronic illnesses trade information and emotional support. During the worst days of the pandemic, social media felt like a lifeline for large swaths of the population as social distancing kept us physically isolated.

Yet despite these benefits (which I'd argue are benefits of the Internet in general, not social media in particular), on balance social platforms are having a net-negative effect on our collective well-being. We're addicted to our phones, our capacity for empathy toward others in online spaces has been reduced, and our need for social approval has been amplified. We're obsessed with status, popularity, appearance. We feel worse about our bodies, and at the same time we feel disembodied, as if we exist in "no place at all," in the words of sociologist and technology scholar Joan Donovan.[27] Some of us have taken to attacking others, both psychologically—trolling and harassing them with weight-based bullying, for instance, on social media[28] and YouTube[29]—and physically, with online hate spilling over into real-world violence. Our trust in science and medicine has eroded. We're experiencing a breakdown of shared truth and repeated threats to democracy.

Many people who helped build major tech platforms and the Internet itself are now speaking out against social media. Numerous Silicon Valley parents (including, famously, Steve Jobs before his death) won't let their own kids use the products they helped create, which are designed to be as addictive as possible. Former Facebook executive (and current billionaire venture capitalist) Chamath Palihapitiya said in a 2017 interview that "the short-term, dopamine-driven feedback loops that we have created [with social media] are destroying how society works."[30] He said that he and others who built Facebook knew deep down that the platform might end up being harmful but went ahead with it anyway. "I feel tremendous guilt," he said. Virtual-reality trail-blazer and tech critic Jaron Lanier, who worked in the 1990s to help the Internet grow to a massive scale, advocates completely disengaging from social platforms in his 2018 book *Ten Arguments for Deleting Your Social Media Accounts Right Now.*[31]

Social media and related technologies have aided and abetted the spread of harmful wellness mis- and disinformation, but they've also done more than that. The platforms *themselves* have undermined our collective well-being. Coupled with Western culture's endemic lack of attention to mental health and social determinants, these technologies have helped create a profoundly unwell society—one that brings out the worst in people and inflames preexisting psychological vulnerabilities and social divisions.

Moreover, there's evidence that these technologies may be doing more to detract from the overall project of social justice than they are to advance it. Engagement-maximizing algorithms have amplified division and hate, and tech companies have failed to act when that was brought to their attention. "We have seen ads on platforms like Facebook violate civil rights laws," said Rashad Robinson, president of the racial-justice organization Color of Change, in 2021 congressional testimony. He spoke of the "near-total control" of Facebook, Amazon, Apple, and Google over online life. "Do not allow the very technology that was supposed to take us into the future to drag us backward and into the past," he implored the U.S. House communications and technology subcommittee.[32]

Social media has connected and increased the reach of overt white supremacists and other bigots who otherwise likely would have remained far more disorganized and been relegated to the fringes. An internal Facebook study in 2016 found that among people who joined extremist groups on the platform, 64 percent did so because Facebook's recommendations algorithms steered them there.[33] In catalyzing extremists, social media also presents a distorted view of public opinion that can reduce the momentum for social change in the real world. In June 2020, just weeks after George Floyd's murder, 70 percent of the most-shared Facebook posts about Black Lives Matter were critical of the movement, even though at the time the majority of American voters were supportive of BLM.[34]

As writer Jenny Odell points out in her 2019 book *How to Do Nothing,* when algorithms constantly hijack our attention and hinder our ability to concentrate at the individual level, it thwarts our capacity for collective concentration and movement-building—for sustaining the attention required to make meaningful change. "In a time that demands action, distraction appears to be (at the level of the collective) a life-and-death matter," she writes.[35]

One of the ways that social media distracts us from these larger concerns is by encouraging compulsive sharing of the most mundane details of our lives, and that's part of what has made wellness culture take off. No matter how small our audiences may be, the very structure of social media rewards us for sharing our workout routines, diet plans, smoothie-bowl recipes, essential-oil "cures," and skin care regimens—the weirder the better, at least from the perspective of the algorithms, because extreme and novel content is grist for the mill of the attention economy. We might only be sharing with a relatively small group of people, but we're still seeing what gets liked and shared, and then adjusting our content—and often our offline behavior—accordingly. We're also helping shape our audiences' feeds and thus their views of the world, because the moment they click "like" on our DIY kombucha recipe, the algorithm nudges them a little bit further into the wilds of wellness culture. We are both the influencers and the influenced.

I'm saying "we" here, but my own status on social media is very different today than it was back when I was just connecting with friends on Friendster, or Myspace, or even in my early days on Facebook. At the time of this writing, I have more than 125,000 people in my audience on Instagram, and more than 15,000 each on Facebook and Twitter. Since beginning to recognize the harm caused by social media I've stopped posting much, but those numbers still make me something of an influencer (though certainly not a "wellness influencer" in the sense of using the platforms to sell supplements and cleanses). I have no doubt that having a large social media audience has helped advance my career in some ways, so I don't want to seem ungrateful, but the truth is that my path to becoming an influencer involved first being influenced by the structure and culture of social media—and not in a way that was good for my mental health, or for my contributions to the discourse.

Despite trying to stick to translating science and specialized information about disordered eating for the general public in a nuanced way, there's only so much subtlety I (or anyone else) can cram into a meme or a caption. What's more, my more polemical posts have been rewarded with likes, shares, and new "followers"—a term I cringe at because of its association with cult leaders, which is increasingly what some influencers can seem like. I've felt social media push me toward more black-and-white ways of writing in my posts, and I know that at times that's translated to less nuanced ways of thinking. I've been pulled into tense comment exchanges and sucked into unwinnable debates. I've spent too many hours and devoted far too much mental space to molehills that loomed like mountains through the lens of social platforms. And I know I'm not alone.

"To me, one of the most troubling ways social media has been used in recent years is to foment waves of hysteria and fear, both by news media and by users themselves," Odell writes. "Whipped into a permanent state of frenzy, people create and subject themselves to news cycles, complaining of anxiety at the same time that they check back ever more diligently."[36]

That state of frenzy is undermining our individual and collective well-being on a day-to-day basis. It's also helping lead some of us down even more dangerous paths, to places where wellness culture and conspiracism intersect.

### Conspirituality

Probably very few people in the wellness world would self-identify as conspiracy theorists, and things like vaccine hesitancy and belief in misinformation can certainly develop for many reasons that have nothing to do with wild theories about government mind control. But today, wellness culture and conspiracy theories are increasingly intertwined. One highly visible symbol of that connection is "QAnon shaman" Jacob Chansley, by far the most recognizable figure among the extremists who stormed the U.S. Capitol on January 6, 2021, with his bare chest, horned fur hat, and painted face, carrying an American flag with a spear on the end. At the time of the insurrection, Chansley, also known as Jake Angeli, was something of an influencer in the world of psychedelics. In 2019 he became a vocal proponent of the QAnon conspiracy theory, and later started showing up at right-wing "Stop the Steal" rallies—held to advocate reinstating Donald Trump to the presidency—before eventually taking part in the storming of the Capitol.

He wasn't the only one from the wellness world who did. Another was Rachel Powell, a yoga and organic-food enthusiast who raised chickens and sold yogurt and cheese at a farmers' market, who was caught in footage of January 6th smashing a window with a battering ram and shouting out orders on a bullhorn. She told *The New Yorker*'s Ronan Farrow that she had a certification as a group fitness instructor and had taken a course in alternative medicine, and a friend described her to Farrow as "very granola, very *crunchy*."[37] Spurred on by misinformation during the pandemic, she refused to obey mask restrictions and attended anti-mask rallies in the months before the Capitol insurrection. She was arrested in February 2021 for her participation in that riot and, charged with multiple felony counts, was released on house arrest pending her trial—on the condition that she wear a mask at all times when in public and be monitored by GPS. In May 2022, she filed a motion asking for the house-arrest order to be overturned because it interfered with her work schedule and ability to raise her children, but her request was denied because of the felony charges and because she had made two violent threats on social media before her arrest. In September 2022, GPS monitoring having proved unenforceable, Powell was ordered held under stricter home confinement.[38]

Chansley, meanwhile, remained in jail ahead of his trial,

and successfully lobbied the correctional facility to provide him only organic food, which he said was necessary for both his religion and his digestion. He also attempted to get released on house arrest because of the increased risk of COVID in the incarcerated population and his refusal to take the vaccine, but that request was denied. The judge said he was too dangerous to be released, in part because Chansley had threatened then–vice president Mike Pence and later told the FBI he was glad he'd done it because Pence was a "child-trafficking traitor"—a talking point emblematic of QAnon. (Chansley has since renounced QAnon, his lawyer told the *New York Times* in late 2021.[39])

What exactly are conspiracy theories, and what distinguishes them from reality?

"Conspiracy theories are attempts to explain the ultimate causes of significant social and political events and circumstances with claims of secret plots by two or more powerful actors," writes a group of researchers led by Karen Douglas, a professor of social psychology at the UK's University of Kent, who has spent many years studying conspiracy theories.[40] "While a conspiracy refers to a true causal chain of events, a conspiracy theory refers to an allegation of conspiracy that may or may not be true." The world has certainly seen its fair share of true conspiracies, health-related and otherwise: the Tuskegee study, the tobacco industry conspiring to deceive the public about the effects of smoking, Watergate. And people have good reason to be wary of conspiracies, particularly if their community has been victim to them in the past. Conspiracy theories also often contain grains of truth, making it easier for people to buy in. But there are some ways of telling the difference between genuine conspiracies and fantastical ones.

A true conspiracy is usually fairly narrow in scope: Richard Nixon and a handful of people in his administration and reelection committee conspired to break into Democratic Party headquarters in order to spy on and sabotage the rival party, and then tried to cover up the crime when they got caught. Conspiracy *theories*, on the other hand, are usually more far-fetched ideas that link together disparate, complex phenomena and don't make a lot of sense—for example, the belief that the government (or is it Bill Gates?) is using COVID vaccines to inject microchip identifiers into everyone, which will also somehow turn people into 5G antennas and/or prevent them from reproducing / kill them. Conspiracy theories often take the form of what French scholars call an "argumentative *mille-feuille*" (*mille-feuille argumentatif*):like those flaky pastries made up of countless thin layers, conspiracy theories consist of details added one on top of the other, giving the impression of a robust explanation that couldn't possibly be entirely wrong.[41] True conspiracies are something altogether different, and they are discovered through what researchers call "conventional thinking"—reasonable skepticism of official accounts, careful consideration of evidence, and a commitment to internal consistency.[42] Genuine conspiracies (and explanations of them) aren't layered with multiple conflicting details, and they aren't presumed to involve a vast global network of bad actors, such as the entire pharmaceutical industry, all conventional doctors, and the governments of multiple countries (as most anti-vaccine conspiracy theorists believe are complicit), even if they do point the finger at a relatively small group.

The psychology of conspiracy theories is complex, but at the most fundamental level, they meet deep inner needs. As Douglas and colleagues explained in a 2017 study, "People appear to be drawn to conspiracy theories when—compared to nonconspiracy explanations—they promise to satisfy important social psychological motives" such as the desire for understanding, certainty, control, security, and positive self-image. In another study, they found that there's a correlation between attachment styles and conspiracy theories: people who have an "anxious" attachment style (marked by a fear of abandonment and deep insecurity in relationships) are more likely to believe in conspiracy theories. As someone who had an anxious attachment style for at least the first three decades of my life, I can identify with what Douglas and her coauthor wrote about the reasons why anxiously attached people might be drawn to conspiracy theories: "anxious attachment predicts low interpersonal trust and increased perceptions of the world as threatening and dangerous, [...so] perhaps endorsement of conspiracy explanations is one way to gain a compensatory feeling of control in an otherwise threatening world filled with untrustworthy others."[43] Douglas cautions that this research is correlational, so we can't infer that attachment styles *cause* people to believe in conspiracy theories. "However, it is difficult to imagine that belief in conspiracy theories changes a person's attachment style," she told me in an email, explaining that attachment style is thought to be relatively unchanging from early childhood onward. (I credit the change in my own attachment style to at least fifteen years of consistent psychotherapy, a privilege that most people unfortunately don't have, followed by more than nine years in a securely attached relationship with a kind and compassionate partner.) "Instead, it makes more sense to argue that attachment styles lead to conspiracy thinking," she says.

If conspiracy theories are a way to gain a sense of control in a threatening world, it's no surprise that they proliferated in the COVID-19 era. In fact, conspiracy theories have been a part of pandemics and epidemics for hundreds of years—at least as far back as the Middle Ages, when conspiracists falsely accused marginalized groups including Jews, Roma, and witches of deliberately spreading bubonic plague.[44] Douglas explains that conspiracy beliefs are stronger when people are living through particularly large-scale or significant events, like pandemics, because in those moments small-scale explanations can seem insufficient. Indeed, when the world is upended and millions of people are dying, the truth that simple tools like vaccines and masks are our best ticket out might feel a little unsatisfying. The existence of a nefarious global cabal poisoning people for profit might somehow seem more fitting given the stakes and scope of the situation. "Conspiracy theories tend to thrive in times of crisis, so I think it is not surprising that we are seeing an uptick in conspiracy theorizing at this time," Douglas told me in early 2021. "People are looking for ways to cope with uncertainty and feelings of powerlessness, and conspiracy theories might seem to offer an explanation, even though it might not be helpful."

That desire to cope with uncertainty is likely part of the reason why, a few months into the pandemic, conspiracy theories started proliferating in wellness spaces. Traditionally, conspiracy theories have often had a largely male audience of hard-core extremists, but in a phenomenon known as pastel QAnon (a reference to the soft and stereotypically feminine aesthetic used in wellness and lifestyle memes), dozens of female wellness and lifestyle influencers with large followings started posting in their Instagram stories and feeds about QAnon and related conspiracy theories. They'd amassed follower counts ranging from the tens of thousands to the millions by posting about wellness topics such as "clean" beauty, yoga, and "natural" parenting, and now suddenly they were making false, outlandish claims about how a major furniture retailer was engaged in child sex trafficking, the pandemic was all a lie, the real scourge was 5G towers, and wearing masks was both ineffective and harmful. They continued to intersperse this conspiracist rhetoric with cheerful messages about self-care and empowerment. Yoga teacher Seane Corn, who was one of the first wellness influencers to speak out against the sudden incursion of QAnon into wellness spaces, told *PBS NewsHour* in early 2022 that she estimates a staggering 50 percent of her inner circle of wellness influencers believes in that conspiracy theory.[45]

How did that happen? The seeds were probably sown years before. Many of these newly conspiracist influencers were already anti-vaccine, which was something of a preexisting condition in wellness spaces, and the anti-vax sentiment ratcheted up as the COVID vaccine became a reality. "In green beauty and wellness, you would be very hard-pressed to find someone who isn't mildly uneasy about vaccines," green beauty influencer and attorney Lola Gusman told *The Lily* in 2021.[46] That pervasive uneasiness made wellness culture a breeding ground for conspiracy theories about vaccines, and numerous studies have found that believing in one conspiracy theory makes people more likely to believe others,[47] which may account for many wellness influencers' sudden adoption of QAnon and other conspiracy theories. "It's incredible how networked these conspiracy theories are," Rachel Moran, a postdoctoral fellow at the University of Washington's Center for an Informed Public who studies disinformation in wellness spaces, told *Mother Jones* in 2022. "Once you're involved in one of the buckets of misinformation, your likelihood to believe in others is far, far amplified."[48]

Take, for example, Christiane Northrup, the OB-GYN turned author and wellness influencer. In 1994 she came out with a book called *Women's Bodies, Women's Wisdom,* and soon she became a regular guest on *Oprah* and *Dr. Oz* and quickly rose to the A-list of wellness influencers (before "influencer" was even a job description). By 2005 an anti-vaccine slant was evident in her work, when she falsely claimed in another book that vaccines could cause a whole host of illnesses. By 2015, she had given up her medical license in the state of Maine (though she continues to use "MD" in her promotional materials) and gone all-in on alternative medicine. And when COVID-19 hit, she quickly slid into promoting conspiracy theories about the virus, inveighing against face masks, and sharing QAnon propaganda, along with increasingly strident anti-vax content.[49]

In 2011, Charlotte Ward, an independent researcher who identifies as a conspiracy theorist, used the term *conspirituality* in the peer-reviewed academic *Journal of Religious Studies* to describe the online phenomenon that saw people with New Age spiritual beliefs and "alternative worldviews" increasingly taken in by conspiracy-like thinking. (The social scientist David Voas, of University College London, a graduate of the London School of Economics and a Cambridge PhD, listed as a coauthor of the now oft-cited paper, was brought on in 2011 to "give [the paper] an academic gloss.")[50] In the decade since the paper was published, conspirituality has exploded. Many conspiracy-theory researchers agree that people in New Age spaces are particularly susceptible to belief in conspiracy theories, in part because, as Douglas and colleagues explain in a 2017 paper, these people "consistently seek patterns and meaning in their environment."[51] Three beliefs common to nearly all conspiracy theories are the ideas that nothing happens by accident, nothing is as it seems, and everything is connected—so people who are primed to seek connections and significance in everyday events are at greater risk of falling into conspiracist thinking.

As far as personality traits go, a propensity for seeking patterns and meaning is largely positive—indeed, it may help foster creativity—but unfortunately, spiritual seekers and "cultural creatives" may be prime targets for conspirituality for this same reason.[52] "I always say that people in the yoga and wellness space already had fertile ground for conspiracy thinking," says Julian Walker, the yoga teacher and cohost of the *Conspirituality* podcast, which chronicles the rise of this type of thinking in contemporary wellness and New Age culture. He explains that there's long been a reflexive reaction among proponents of alternative medicine whenever they encounter skepticism: "They'll very quickly give you a conspiracy kind of explanation, even though they won't call it a conspiracy—they'll say, 'well, there's no funding for that research because Big Pharma doesn't want you to take away from their profits.'" (That's a common line of rhetoric in wellness culture, but it's actually misleading and the product of what Walker calls "an excellent PR job" by advocates of complementary and alternative medicine, as we'll discuss in Chapter 6.)

Moreover, some experts who study conspiracy theories say another trait that may make people in the wellness community susceptible is the tendency to rely more heavily on intuition than on analytical thinking. Again, being an intuitive thinker can be helpful in certain areas of life—I know from personal experience, having spent more than a decade practicing and teaching intuitive eating. For those of us who tend to overintellectualize, learning to tap into intuition and the mind-body connection can be revelatory not just for eating but also for other aspects of self-care and decision-making. For one thing, "trusting your gut" can help you know when a relationship or other interpersonal situation just doesn't feel right. Yet relying too much on intuition in all areas of life, at the expense of critical thinking, can make us susceptible to mis- and disinformation. "When we are forced to be extremely independent and discerning when it comes to our health, it is understandable why some people follow that thread and become alarmed about everything—their water, air, microwaves. And then vaccines. And then COVID. And then masks," wrote clean-beauty brand director Merrady Wickes on Instagram a week after the January 6 insurrection. "Being involved in wellness and green/clean beauty leaves you vulnerable to distrusting everything and everyone."[53]

Indeed, spending time in wellness spaces tends to expose people to more conspiracy theories. A 2021 report by researchers from George Washington University's Institute for Data, Democracy & Politics found that online alternative-health communities such as Facebook parenting groups dedicated to homeopathy, naturopathy, and spiritual healing "act as the critical conduits between conspiracy theorists and parents."[54] These groups are where conspiracy theories get watered down, painted in pastels, and repackaged in ways that make them more palatable to people who are closer to the mainstream, who might not otherwise give those theories serious consideration. This repackaging can happen even in relatively small groups, which Facebook doesn't tend to moderate, even though they're major channels for misinformation.

The link between alternative medicine and conspiracy theories also goes beyond online groups. A 2014 University of Chicago study about conspiracy beliefs found that a staggering 49 percent of Americans believe in at least one medical conspiracy theory, and 18 percent believe in three or more.[55] Many of us, or our friends and family, might be part of those groups. The Chicago study also found that there was a link between the use of alternative medicine (especially *instead* of conventional medicine) and belief in any medical conspiracy theory, and that people who believed in three or more of these theories were more likely to buy organic or farmers'-market foods and use herbal supplements than those who believed in fewer. There's nothing wrong with organic foods or farmers' markets, of course—it's the conspiracy theories that are the problem, and "crunchy" interests can unfortunately sometimes put people directly in the path of the misinformation firehose.

That may be partly by design—and not just the design of the algorithms. Of course it's hard to know which came first, conspiracy beliefs or the use of alternative medicine, but for marketing purposes it's not a bad bet for the makers of wellness-culture products and programs to seed and feed conspiracist fears. We see that in the clean-beauty line that says, "The FDA only bans 11 toxic ingredients; we've banned 1,500." Or the complementary and alternative medicine practitioners using outlandish claims about "Big Pharma, the government, and the media" to sell an expensive "vaccine detox" protocol. Or the organic grocery-delivery service claiming that products labeled as organic in other grocery stores probably aren't—and that the only way to ensure you're getting *truly* organic food is to sign up for their service. Conspiracy theories whip up fear, and fear sells. That may be a key part of why the wellness industry has ballooned into a multitrillion-dollar business in recent years. As medical doctor and wellness critic Jen Gunter wrote in 2018, "there can be no modern wellness industry without medical conspiracy theories."[56]

There could also be no modern wellness industry without the fetishization and appropriation of non-Western cultures, as we've discussed—and the conspiritualist strain of wellness culture commonly engages in this appropriation, too, particularly with South and East Asian cultures. *Vox* reporter Terry Nguyen cites the example of a holistic facialist in Miami Beach, who posted on Instagram in 2021 that wearing a mask blocks the flow of "Lung Qi," a term from traditional Chinese medicine meaning "energy." This false claim, Nguyen writes, is "a type of medical Orientalism that exoticizes non-Western practices and caters to New Age notions of mystical, 'natural' healing."[57] It also helps obscure the antisocial nature of refusing to wear a mask, wrapping it in the false flag of cultural tradition. What's more, traditional Chinese medicine hasn't been a bastion of conspirituality during the pandemic the way other types of complementary and alternative medicine have, as Walker and his *Conspirituality* cohosts pointed out in 2022.[58]

Many of us might think we're impervious to conspiracy theories (wellness related and otherwise), and some of us would be right. As individuals, we may not all be equally likely to buy into conspiracism; spiritual or creative types who tend to seek out meaning and connections between disparate phenomena might be more vulnerable. But at the collective level, conspiracy theories can harm us all—as is the case with the ones at the heart of the anti-vaccine movement, which we'll discuss next.

# CHAPTER 5

# The Anti-Vax Rabbit Hole

Growing up, Anita Emly had a somewhat complicated relationship with Western medicine. Her father generally dismissed it, turning instead to alternative treatments from his homeland of India, from which he'd immigrated to New York City before Emly was born. "He had an herbal thing for anything, whether it was clove or turmeric or this ginger thing he made when you had a cold," she says—and this was in the 1980s and '90s, when herbs and alternative medicine were nowhere near as mainstream as they are today. Her mother, who is from Puerto Rico, stuck to conventional treatments like Tylenol, but she didn't completely trust doctors—likely because, Emly says, she'd had her own experience of complaints being dismissed or minimized. Her father initially thought that vaccinating their kids was unnecessary, but he changed his tune after learning it was mandatory for school enrollment. But Emly says her mother later revealed that if she'd been in a different position—more at home in the city, more fluent in English, more financially secure—she might have decided to home-school her kids, and thus would have avoided having to vaccinate them. As it was, Emly got all her childhood immunizations. She produced proof of vaccination to the college she attended, and later went on to get the vaccines necessary to study abroad, although she was always a little hesitant. "I remember being nervous, but not about anything in particular," she says. "Just like, 'it's an injection, what does it do? Am I going to have a bad reaction to it?'"

It wasn't until she was about to become a mom herself that this long-standing hesitancy coalesced into something more concrete, and more harmful. Pregnant with her first child and hungry for information about how to raise a healthy baby, she was directed by a trusted coworker to a popular but problematic parenting book that grossly inflates the risk posed by vaccines and minimizes the risk of vaccine-preventable diseases.[1] "My coworker was very educated," she says. "He had a Ph.D.—not anything related to vaccines, but he was an educated person and he recommended [this] book, so I kind of thought I was in safe territory." Unfortunately, she was not. Like many new parents and parents-to-be, her efforts to do the best for her child would soon expose her to a whole world of wellness misinformation.

She started fretting over the safety of the ingredients in vaccines, and online research led her to dubious sources that at the time she didn't know were problematic. When she began talking to her friends about vaccines, she learned that many of them weren't planning on vaccinating their kids. In their group—a religious Christian community, with friends involved in various churches across the country, who all stayed in touch on Facebook—not vaccinating was seen as a valid parenting choice, similar to different sleep philosophies or feeding practices. There was a vibe of trying not to judge each other's choices, so she saw a lot of anti-vaccine content in her Facebook feed without much pushback.

After her daughter was born, Emly started refusing some of the vaccines on the standard schedule, and then eventually stopped having her daughter vaccinated altogether. She never actually saw herself as *anti*-vaccine, though—especially compared to others in her life. "I have loved ones who are ferociously anti-vaccine and think that vaccines should never be used for anything," she says. "And so because I wasn't, like, militantly anti-vaccine, I didn't think I was anti-vaccine—even though my daughter was very under-vaccinated and I stopped vaccinating her at age one." In a community where anti-vax sentiment was the norm, the fact that Emly had allowed her daughter to get *any* immunizations at all seemed balanced. Now an advocate for vaccination, she recognizes that her skepticism of Western medicine, lack of understanding of vaccine science, and preexisting anxiety about vaccines, along with the attitudes in her community, created fertile ground for her to develop what were for all intents and purposes anti-vax behaviors. "I was like, 'I'm not anti-vaccine, I'm just looking at the risks and benefits, and I'm deciding that sometimes the risks outweigh the benefits'— based on faulty information," she says.

The world of wellness is rife with distortions, half-truths, and outright scams, but perhaps no form of wellness misinformation is more harmful than the anti-vaccine movement, which can have deadly consequences not only for the person who buys into it but also for anyone else in their orbit. And unfortunately, it seems that more and more people in the wellness world are getting sucked in. Anti-vax accounts saw staggering growth on social media during the pandemic, adding 10.1 million followers across platforms in 2020 to reach a total English-language audience of 59.2 million people—and alternative-health entrepreneurs are responsible for nearly 40 percent of that following, according to a report from the tech watchdog group Center for Countering Digital Hate (CCDH), which studies misinformation and hate speech.[2] The CCDH dubbed twelve leading anti-vax influencers "the Disinformation Dozen" because it found that they were responsible for 65 percent or more of online anti-vaccine content, and among them are many prominent wellness influencers: Joseph Mercola, a wellness entrepreneur whom the *New York Times* called "the most influential spreader of COVID-19 misinformation online"; Christiane Northrup, the medical doctor turned wellness entrepreneur and alternative-medicine advocate, who began spreading COVID conspiracy theories early in the pandemic and was very influential in helping them move out of QAnon groups and into mainstream social media spaces; Sayer Ji, who runs a popular alternative-health website and related social media accounts that promote baseless wellness claims and anti-vaccine misinformation; and Kelly Brogan, the "holistic psychiatrist" and former *goop* contributor we discussed in Chapter 3 (who was married to Ji until 2022), who encouraged her followers not to wear masks during the pandemic and claimed early on that "there is potentially no such thing as the coronavirus."[3]

These wellness entrepreneurs, and many others, have made millions promoting and selling unproven remedies for COVID and other diseases for which vaccines are available and recommended, as well as "detoxes" to supposedly cleanse the body if you have been vaccinated. Tech platforms were slow to step in and remove the harmful claims, failing to act on 95 percent of the COVID and vaccine misinformation reported to them, according to a 2020 CCDH report—likely because, according to the organization's calculations, social media companies were pulling in a billion dollars a year in ad revenue from anti-vaccine misinformation.[4]

Wild misconceptions about the COVID vaccine multiplied on social media, like the conspiracy-theory video released in May 2020 that falsely claimed the novel coronavirus was deliberately engineered in order to bring profit to global elites. That video was watched millions of times—and got more engagement on Facebook than videos with far more mainstream appeal, like the one where the cast of *The Office* reunited for a Zoom wedding, or Taylor Swift's exclusively online concert—before finally being removed by major social media companies and video-sharing platforms for violating their terms of service.[5] The video had initially gained traction after being shared in a Facebook group dedicated to QAnon, and then spread by Christiane Northrup.

Of course not all wellness entrepreneurs and practitioners are anti-vaccine, anti-mask, QAnon supporters. Many wellness influencers used their platforms to urge people to mask up, get vaccinated, and practice other sensible public health measures. Still, anti-vax views are strikingly prevalent in the wellness world, which is due in part to the fact that one of the core values of wellness culture is the mistrust of mainstream medicine. Social media algorithms have also done much to amplify anti-vax and conspiratorial views.

To understand how all these forms of misinformation intersect in the wellness space, and what we can do to stop their spread, it's helpful to look at how and why people come to believe them—and how some are able to rethink their views.

### The Gateway Effect

Like many new moms in San Francisco, when Renée DiResta gave birth to her first child, she started doing some things that could be considered wellness-y, like making her own baby food and using cloth diapers. Because she'd expressed interest in those things, Facebook's algorithm pegged her as a "crunchy" parent. "I'm really not, which is funny, but [the algorithm] inferred that I am," she says. "And so then it started to show me other things that crunchy people like," such as backyard chicken raising ("a joy, except for the photos of chicken ailments"), organic products—and anti-vaccine groups. Lots of them. The one that the algorithm pushed to her most aggressively seemed to have Facebook as a central part of its growth strategy: Group leaders launched a GoFundMe campaign and raised $10,000 to run paid Facebook ads targeting new parents with reports of sudden infant death that the leaders claimed was caused by vaccines.

For too many people, harmless wellness-culture pursuits like cloth diapering or an interest in backyard chickens can be a gateway into destructive forms of misinformation. It's a continuum, and in some cases a slippery slope: People get pulled in by the cute chickens or the promise of less diaper rash for their baby, and along the way they start to adopt anti-establishment views about wellness or deepen preexisting ones. That skeptical stance in some cases then leads, via the machinery of social media and targeted advertising, to more and more far-fetched beliefs and more and more unproven cures. I've slid a ways down that slope myself in the past, and I know how it is: You're trying to do the best you can to take care of yourself and/or your family, and conventional medicine hasn't been much help, so you start "doing your research" and suddenly you're down the rabbit hole.

DiResta, for her part, was disturbed by the algorithm's targeting her with anti-vax content. Perhaps because she was *not* actually the crunchy mom that Facebook assumed her to be, she questioned those recommendations and eventually started looking into why these anti-vaccine groups were proliferating on social media. She worked in the tech field at the time, and she began researching how online anti-vax content was influencing offline trends. It was around the time of the measles outbreak at Disneyland in 2014–2015 that produced nearly 150 cases in multiple states,[6] and outbreaks were occurring in other places, too. Public health officials were alarmed by the resurgence of this vaccine-preventable disease, which had been declared eliminated from the U.S. in 2000, thanks to a robust vaccination program.[7] But that didn't last long. According to the CDC, in 2019 the country had 1,274 confirmed cases of measles in thirty-one states—the greatest number of cases reported in the U.S. since 1992.[8] The majority of those cases were in people who weren't vaccinated against the disease—adults or, in some cases, very young children not yet due for the vaccine. The 2019 figure mirrored a 30 percent increase in measles cases worldwide the same year, prompting the World Health Organization (WHO) to declare vaccine hesitancy one of the top ten global threats.[9]

Many anti-vaccine adherents are just trying to do what's safest for their kids and families, and yet their refusal to vaccinate is having the opposite effect—not only for them, but for millions of other people as well.

Following the 2014–2015 uptick in measles cases, several states began to introduce bills to ban vaccine exemptions based on so-called personal beliefs. DiResta cofounded an organization called Vaccinate California to push for such legislation in her home state. That's when she realized that "anti-vax Twitter" was using the platform to create the illusion of overwhelming opposition to vaccines and her group's bill. Movement leaders would ask their followers to tweet at state assembly representatives to let them know that voting in favor of the bill would be a career killer. "Since anti-vax activists lose on the science and are small in number, they have increasingly begun to rely on social media to inflate their presence," DiResta wrote in 2015.[10] "The goal of anti-vax Twitter is to dominate the conversation and make it look as if all parents are vehemently opposed to the legislation." Anti-vax Twitter also underwent what DiResta calls "an evolution in messaging," where the movement discovered that focusing on arguments about personal freedom and "vaccine choice" was more effective than focusing on autism and toxins, as they had been doing for years.[11]

Although there's been opposition to vaccines for as long as they've existed—in the late 1790s, the first anti-vaccine advocates argued that the smallpox inoculation (made from the fluid in cowpox sores) could cause its recipients to sprout cow horns and develop ox-like features[12]—the modern-day anti-vax movement can be traced back to 1998. That's when Andrew Wakefield (who in 2010 lost his medical license for committing "serious professional misconduct" including dishonesty and ethical violations) published, with twelve coauthors, an explosive study purporting to link the MMR vaccine to autism. The paper was ostensibly a case report of twelve children—an extremely small sample size, and not the kind of research that can tell you anything about causation. It reported that eight of its subjects had developed "behavioural symptoms" days after receiving the MMR vaccine. In fact, it later was revealed that in many instances the symptoms actually appeared either before or months after the children received the vaccines. Wakefield had fudged the timeline to make it seem that the inoculation was the culprit.[13]

Wakefield's article was published in *The Lancet*, one of the most reputable scientific journals in the world. The publication's editors had known that the paper was a bombshell, and they'd proceeded with caution, sending it to four specialists for peer review and conducting three editorial committee meetings to discuss it.[14] During that process, some reviewers were critical, pointing to the small sample size and to the obvious fact that the study design was not randomized or controlled. But rather than simply decline to publish the paper, the journal decided to run it alongside a highly skeptical commentary.[15] The article itself included cautious language of the kind that scientific papers are supposed to use, acknowledging that the link wasn't definitive and that more research was needed. But Wakefield took a very different tone in interviews with the media. In a press conference that an attendee later called "one of the biggest public relations disasters in medicine,"[16] Wakefield exhibited a striking level of certainty for someone whose study only included twelve people, telling journalists that parents should dramatically slow down and space out their children's vaccinations, and that as "a moral issue" he could no longer support the use of the MMR vaccine.[17]

What he didn't tell them was that before the paper was published, he had filed for two patents: one for a new method of diagnosing Crohn's disease by first detecting the measles virus, and the second for an alternative, supposedly "safer" measles vaccine.[18] As journalist Anna Merlan reported in her 2019 book *Republic of Lies*, "Wakefield expected that the test for diagnosing Crohn's could bring in 28 million Euros in revenue, according to a prospectus he created for potential investors, much of that coming from 'litigation-driven testing' of patients in the United States and Britain."[19] He also didn't tell the assembled journalists at the press conference that half the children in the case report were already involved in a lawsuit looking into the effects of the MMR vaccine—a lawsuit for which he himself was a consultant who'd been paid hundreds of thousands of dollars.[20] The parents of some of the children who had developed symptoms of autism before being vaccinated changed their stories after getting involved with the lawsuit. These details make it clear that the results of his study were a foregone conclusion, not science at all. Those conflicts of interest, in addition to a number of other ethical violations related to the 1998 paper, eventually caused *The Lancet* to retract the paper and Wakefield to lose his medical license in 2010. But by then, the damage had already been done.

Instead of digging around and finding the inconsistencies in Wakefield's paper, nearly all of the journalists who'd attended that press conference published relatively uncritical stories about his study the following day, and you can probably guess what happened next: a media frenzy, causing UK vaccination rates to take a nosedive in the following years. Places in England where more than 90 percent of children had been vaccinated before Wakefield's study saw their immunization rates drop precipitously to less than 70 percent, far short of the numbers needed for herd immunity.[21] Measles subsequently reached epidemic levels in England and Wales. The British media continued reporting on the study for several years, with coverage peaking between 2001 and 2003. The panic spread to the United States, where TV personality Jenny McCarthy took up the cause. McCarthy's son's diagnosis of autism and her popular platform on ABC's *The View* made her the unofficial spokeswoman for doubts about the MMR vaccine. Oprah, Larry King, and *People* magazine positioned McCarthy as an expert on autism, abetting her anti-vax campaign.[22]

The U.S. subsequently became the hub of the anti-vax movement, which experts say is no coincidence. The private, for-profit American healthcare system often raises suspicion (in some cases rightly) that pharmaceutical companies are simply out to make money and not to help the public good, which makes the U.S. fertile ground for conspiracy theories about vaccines and healthcare in general. Although the wellness industry is also clearly motivated by profit, that's not as widely understood or discussed as the role of "Big Pharma," which is routinely decried by anti-vaxxers and wellness culture more broadly.

Andrew Wakefield moved to the U.S. in 2004, making his new home in Austin, Texas, where for six years he directed a clinic that studied developmental disorders in children. (He was not licensed to practice medicine in the United States.) He left the clinic in 2010, after losing his UK medical license.[23]

Despite having had his theory disproven, his article retracted from the *Lancet*, and his license revoked, Wakefield is still pushing his anti-vaccine views, with all their inherent ableism. He treats autism as a horrible scourge, whose existence is supposedly caused by toxins from the MMR vaccine getting into the brain and damaging it. Food and a "leaky gut" are somehow also involved (we'll discuss the problems with the "leaky gut" label in the next chapter).

That's Wakefield's new thing—he's now peddling claims about "gut health" and gluten-free diets as the key to preventing and reversing autism, despite no sound evidence. A review of the literature in 2013 evaluating the use of gluten-free diets in people with autism found that they provided no benefit,[24] and numerous studies since then have found no improvement in behavioral or bowel symptoms in kids with autism on gluten-free diets or diets free of both gluten and casein (the protein in milk). For example, a 2021 literature review found that the available evidence doesn't show any benefit of a gluten-free diet for people on the autism spectrum who don't *also* have a clinical diagnosis of celiac disease (a genetic condition that creates an intolerance to gluten and affects 1 percent or less of the population).[25] Yet Wakefield and other peddlers of wellness misinformation continue to insist upon the benefits of these dietary changes for everyone with autism. These wellness-diet ideas coexist with Wakefield's anti-vax views; neither went away when he lost his credentials. Indeed, his diet advice is part of the often swift progression from wellness culture to the anti-vax movement. "A lot of parents with autistic kids who go down the anti-vaccine road start by restrictive diets," Merlan said in a 2020 interview for the podcast *The Dream.* "It is a totally understandable thing to want to cut something out of your kid's diet that you think might be hurting them, and it is sort of a gateway toward some of these other claims."[26]

Just as wellness can be an entry point to anti-vaccine views, the reverse can also happen. "I think being anti-vaccine deepened my ventures into wellness, because you feel like, 'if I don't want to use vaccines to protect my kid, what can I do?'" Emly says. "I think anti-vaccine was my kind of gateway into all of that, because I did want to boost their immune system and protect them from toxins," she says. With that goal in mind, she "did her own research"— a common phrase among anti-vax adherents that means, essentially, to immerse yourself in the vaccine-related content suggested by algorithms and anti-vax groups—and found misinformation that made her fearful of all kinds of chemicals, from household cleaners to foods and medicines. "The idea of 'the dose makes the poison' was nowhere on my radar," she says. "I didn't even want to give my kid a non-organic apple." During flu season, in lieu of getting the flu shot, she and her family took supplements and tinctures that she believed would help boost their immune system and ward off illness.

The fact that some people in the anti-vax world tend to slide deeper into wellness culture may be part of the reason Wakefield has pivoted to selling wellness-diet products and programs: clearly there's a market for them.

## Misinformation Superhighways

To some within the anti-vaccine movement, it can feel like an incredible community of like-minded people who've spontaneously connected online and started sharing helpful information. So it may not be obvious that there's a whole machinery designed to push the anti-vax agenda. "When you're in the midst of it, it just feels organic," Emly says. "It doesn't seem like there's this organized campaign to persuade—it feels more grassroots. It doesn't feel like you're targeted as much as you are." Heather Simpson, a mom and former anti-vax influencer turned pro-vaccine advocate, agrees. She was introduced to the anti-vax world in 2015, but it wasn't until early 2019 that she posted her first "vaccine-hesitant" sentiment on Facebook (she'd deliberately toned it down because she was nervous to come out as fully anti-vax). The post blew up—she estimates it was shared a thousand times—and she started getting friend requests from other anti-vaxxers. Hundreds of them. "The friend requests were pouring in, like ten friend requests per minute," she says. But it didn't just feel like the result of one viral post; to her it seemed like the whole anti-vax community was experiencing massive, organic growth all at the same time. "We all filled up our five-thousand-friends lists within like a month," she says. "It was so odd. All of us found each other at one time."

Now, with hindsight and a more critical eye, both Simpson and Emly see that this community is anything but grassroots. According to Imran Ahmed, the founder and CEO of the CCDH and a member of the UK government's independent Commission for Countering Extremism Pilot task force steering committee (no longer active),[27] the big names in the anti-vax space are sophisticated operators who often have dozens of employees. These companies know exactly what they're doing, and to them it's big business. Many of them have contractors overseas who do A/B testing on all of their content to determine the most effective ways to target people with the anti-vax message. Some Disinformation Dozen members, recognizing the even greater lack of moderation of Spanish-language content on social media platforms, had their anti-vax content translated and pumped out to Spanish-speaking communities. And they do all of this high-level manipulation in a way that's designed to be imperceptible to the average audience member. "Anti-vaccine messaging always seems to have a sales pitch on it, but I never noticed that at the time," Emly says. "You know, 'don't trust the flu vaccine, but here, buy this elderberry tonic.'"

Simpson's first foray into the anti-vax world was through a sales pitch, when she was targeted in a 2015 Facebook ad campaign for an anti-vax docuseries. The ads were very persuasive, with a sense of urgency—"this is the only time you'll ever get to watch it, so sign up right now"—and promised to share hidden secrets about vaccines that anyone who cared about their kids needed to read. Simpson didn't have a child yet at the time, but she was planning to and was eager to get a jump on her parenting education. Wanting not to miss her chance to see this "essential" information, she shelled out $200 for the series, and that's how she fell into the trap. Later, she says, when she was an anti-vax influencer herself, a prominent activist—who was the second-biggest anti-vax advertiser on Facebook before he got kicked off, and who bills himself as a "healthy lifestyle advocate"—approached her about working together. She says he told her that he was an affiliate for the docuseries (meaning he received a cut of all the sales that came through his advertising efforts), and that he'd made $40,000 in a single campaign. Simpson says she didn't end up working with him because he rubbed her the wrong way, but she shares this story now because "it opens people's eyes to see how it is kind of about money for some of these people."

Perhaps unsurprisingly, anti-vax targeting and pitching reached a new level during the COVID-19 pandemic, which was a prime situation for what philosophers call "epistemic anxiety"—

a state of uncertainty in which it's hard to know if, when, or how your questions might get answered. "People are more vulnerable when they're in a state of epistemic anxiety," Ahmed said in a 2021 webinar hosted by the Center for Humane Technology.[28] "[Anti-vaccine entrepreneurs] know that, and that's when they go in. It's a sales industry which finds people in a moment of vulnerability and sells them misinformation." That was true before the pandemic, when these entrepreneurs would target anxious moms-to-be and grieving parents, but COVID-19 ratcheted it up to new levels. DiResta, who is now the research manager at Stanford Internet Observatory, wrote an article for *The Atlantic* in 2020 headlined "Anti-vaxxers Think This Is Their Moment." In it she described how some leaders of the anti-vaccine movement deliberately and intentionally used the uncertainty of the pandemic to spread and profit from vaccine misinformation.[29]

Smaller platforms such as Telegram and Parler have encouraged anti-vax content through their lack of moderation, but major tech companies did eventually crack down on misinformation about the COVID vaccine—yet by then it was too little, too late. For example, in October of 2020, YouTube announced that going forward it would ban any videos that contained information about COVID-19 vaccines that contradicted consensus from health authorities including the World Health Organization.[30] The platform told Reuters that this would include removing videos claiming that vaccines kill people or cause infertility, or that microchips would be implanted in people who receive the vaccine. But a YouTube spokesman said that videos containing general discussions about "broad concerns" over the vaccine would be allowed to remain on the platform, and it took until September of 2021 for YouTube to ban several major anti-vax entrepreneurs including the osteopathic physician Joseph Mercola; Mercola's girlfriend Erin Elizabeth, of the blog "Health Nut News"; and Robert F. Kennedy Jr.[31] Similarly, in December of 2020, Twitter announced that it would start removing tweets that spread misinformation about COVID vaccines and would begin labeling tweets that promote conspiracy theories, and the plat-form—along with Facebook, Instagram, and YouTube—devel-oped stricter policies against anti-vax content than it had earlier in the pandemic. Yet as of this writing in October of 2022, Mer-cola's Twitter account still includes links to anti-vaccine content. One of his workarounds is writing random, non-vaccine-related text in the body of the tweet ("Here's what curcumin can do for your health"[32]), seemingly to evade the platform's efforts at auto-mated moderation. Another is the use of sarcasm—posting a photo of CDC director Rochelle Walensky getting a COVID booster shot, Mercola tweeted: "If it's been more than 2 months, time for the latest jab – and get your flu jab. That's why God gave you two arms!"[33] He has also moved some of his content to Sub-stack. Meanwhile, Meta (the parent company of Facebook and Instagram) has banned Kennedy's anti-vax organization, Chil-dren's Health Defense, but its enforcement against Kennedy and his company has been scattershot: though his personal Insta-gram account was banned in February 2021, his public Facebook page, with 344,000 followers, was still active as of October 2022.[34]

Part of the major social media companies' slowness in respond-ing to anti-vax content likely has to do with the fact that such action required creating checks on their own algorithms, which inadvertently favor misinformation. "If you're an ordinary person who's having doubts about the vaccine and you start looking for answers, you're far more likely to come across an anti-vax source than you are an authoritative source like the NHS [National Health Service] or CDC," Callum Hood of the CCDH told the *Guardian*.[35] Algorithms that pick up on some vaccine hesitancy ultimately channel people down the anti-vax rabbit hole. A 2021 report by the CCDH explains that when staffers created new Insta-gram user profiles and followed a variety of different accounts, the ones following a mix of conspiracy accounts and health authori-ties (such as the CDC) were given recommendations for additional misinformation about COVID and vaccines.[36] The only users who *didn't* receive misinformation recommendations were the ones who strictly followed health authorities and not a single conspiracy account. And once people start getting exposed to anti-vax misinformation, they may begin posting vaccine-hesitant or anti-vaccine sentiments themselves, causing the algorithms to funnel new followers to them—a kind of social reinforcement that helps to cement their anti-vax views. "These are effective and very intentional ways of radicalizing people," Hood said.

The problem is not just the algorithms; bad actors also harness social media to spread false information. This is classic disinformation, where the actors are knowingly telling lies. A 2018 study in the *American Journal of Public Health* found that some of the same Russian disinformation accounts that had been used to sow political discord during the 2016 election had turned their attention to vaccines, in an effort to create and inflame divisions around the issue.[37] The study found that both Russian trolls (real people who create and use fake social media accounts for destructive purposes) and bots (automated social media accounts programmed to share misinformation) are significantly more likely to tweet about vaccination than average Twitter users. Interestingly, the behavior of bots and trolls differs: Bots tend to disseminate straightforwardly anti-vaccine messages, whereas trolls promote both pro- and anti-vaccine content, in an effort to sow chaos and undermine democracy. (This technique isn't unique to vaccine tweets; Russian trolls are known to post on both sides of many other divisive issues as well.) Both of these types of accounts pose as everyday users on the platform in order to create the false sense that the anti-vaccine movement is larger and the debate about vaccines is louder than it really is, with the aim of eroding public consensus on vaccination.

Anti-vax views can be found across the political spectrum, but they seem to be increasingly common on the right, even though historically the "crunchy" folks to whom anti-vax groups were marketed often tended to be left-leaning. A lot of that shift likely has to do with Donald Trump, who has opposed vaccines since at least 2014 and was the first American president to be on record as having anti-vaccine views.[38] (He did, however, get vaccinated against COVID-19, which enraged his anti-vax base.) Right-wing conspiracy theorist Alex Jones also helped fan the flames, especially since the start of the pandemic. Gallup polls have found that the percentage of Republicans who say it is either extremely or very important for parents to vaccinate their children has steadily declined over the years, from 93 percent in 2001 to only 79 percent in 2019. In those same years the percentages for Democrats also declined, but less so, going from 97 percent to 92 percent.[39] A March 2021 poll found that white Republicans were more likely to reject the COVID-19 vaccine than any other subset of Americans.[40]

Meanwhile, Black, Indigenous, and Latino communities were specifically targeted with anti-vax rhetoric during the pandemic, despite the fact that these groups were disproportionately impacted by the virus.[41] Marginalized communities have long been the target of anti-vaccination activists and their misinformation campaigns. Children's Health Defense, founded by Robert F. Kennedy Jr., released an hourlong film in March 2021 promoting false claims that COVID-19 vaccination efforts are "part of a larger, sinister experiment on Black communities," invoking the specter of the Tuskegee study, *NBC News* reported.[42] Religious minorities are targets of misinformation, too, particularly sensationalized reports of the use of pork products in vaccines. While pork-derived gelatin is used as a stabilizer in many vaccines, spokespeople for Pfizer, Moderna, and AstraZeneca told *ABC News* in 2020 that their COVID-19 vaccines contain no pork products. Moreover, religious law has adapted to address this concern, "especially when we are concerned about sicknesses," said Rabbi David Stav, chairman of a rabbinical organization in Israel. When it comes to pork gelatin in vaccines, "there is no prohibition and no problem."[43] Similarly, many Islamic authorities around the world have said that the COVID vaccine would be permitted even if it did contain pork products.

Women are another major target of anti-vax misinformation, perhaps because they tend to be in charge of the health-related decisions for their families, including the decision to vaccinate. In 2015, a group of researchers analyzed 800 vaccine-related posts on Pinterest, whose users are overwhelmingly women, and found that 74 percent of those posts were anti-vaccine.[44] In the early days of COVID-19 vaccination, women of childbearing age were targeted on social media with unfounded but scientific-sounding claims that the vaccines could decrease fertility or result in the loss of a pregnancy, leading even some doctors and nurses to express fear. For example, Niharika Sathe, an internal medicine physician in New Jersey, told the *Washington Post* that she first heard the fertility rumor from another doctor, who said she was planning to decline the vaccine for that reason.[45] Sathe, who was pregnant at the time, ended up doing a deep dive into the research and determined that the rumor was false, and both she and her friend got vaccinated after all. But the experience left her shaken. "That kind of misinformation is really scary," she said. "It has enough science to sound potentially plausible." Thanks in large part to false rumors spread about the vaccine on social media, women in their childbearing years were one of the most vaccine-hesitant groups in early 2021, even though the evidence was already clear that if you were pregnant and contracted COVID-19, you were likely to have a more severe case than a non-pregnant woman the same age. Infection with COVID-19 during pregnancy is also associated with an increased risk of preterm birth, and the WHO recommended vaccination for pregnant women "whenever there is risk of the disease." Pregnant people were, in short, a high-priority group to get the vaccine.[46]

Since well before COVID, one of the primary pools from which the anti-vax movement has recruited members is mothers who've lost a baby. In 2019 alone, according to *NBC News*, the host of one of the largest and most active anti-vax groups on Facebook published more than twenty different articles claiming that babies had died from vaccinations—even though coroners in those cases ruled that the deaths had nothing to do with vaccines but instead resulted from sudden infant death syndrome, pneumonia, accidental asphyxiation, or one of a range of other causes.[47] In at least two cases, the asphyxiation was attributed to co-sleeping with a parent. As a mom of an infant myself, I can only imagine how unspeakably heartbreaking it must be to lose a child, particularly in cases where the death was sudden and unexpected. Official reports on both of those asphyxiation cases show that initially the parents seemed to feel responsible for the deaths, saying things like "this is because she was sleeping with me." The pain they felt must have been crushing. But soon both mothers were drawn into the anti-vaccine community on Facebook and began pointing a finger at vaccines instead. In situations of such extreme grief, it's understandable to look for an external cause, rather than to descend into a pit of despair and self-condemnation. But the anti-vax movement swoops in just when these parents are at their most vulnerable, selling them the lie that vaccines are literal poison. Other parents online witness this rhetoric, and those who haven't lost a child become terrified that they will. "In my head I was thinking, if my kid gets a shot, she will die," Heather Simpson says. "I was absolutely convinced. The words 'vaccine' and 'death' were interchangeable in my mind."

### Inoculation

Anita Emly's anti-vaccine views started to evolve when several people close to her got the flu. Her two-year-old, who was still breastfeeding at the time, got sick first. Initially Emly wasn't worried, as she believed that the immune-system benefits conferred by breast milk would protect her daughter from getting too sick. But a few days into the illness, the child's fever reached a staggering 106 degrees and she wouldn't nurse or even open her eyes; she just whimpered and uttered weak cries. Emly rushed her to the doctor, who was able to bring down her fever and diagnosed her with influenza A. Soon after that, Emly and her husband both fell ill.

Her mother and aunt offered to come over and take care of them, but initially Emly told them to keep their distance. "She and her sister are senior citizens, have multiple chronic conditions, and eat highly processed diets," Emly wrote in a 2020 blog post. "If the flu was knocking us down for the count (two healthy thirty-somethings), I was afraid of what it would do to them."[48] Undeterred, her mother and aunt let themselves in with the Emlys' house key, and the two older women helped nurse the young family back to health. Emly thought she would need to return the favor when her mom and aunt got sick, but that never happened. They both had had their flu shots, and they didn't contract the virus—even after spending days in close quarters with three flu-ridden people.

Looking back now, Emly recognizes that that was the first major crack in the wall of her anti-vax beliefs. But as is often the case when something challenges our deeply held views and sense of identity, change doesn't happen overnight. "That experience with my daughter and my mom and aunt got me to be like, wow, okay, the vaccine is really powerful and really effective," Emly says, "but it didn't take away the fear that I had that was already very ingrained." In her mental pro-con list, the experience was a major point in favor of vaccines, but it didn't outweigh what she believed were the cons.

Being willing to rethink your own views in the face of evidence can make it easier to eventually break free from misinformation, as Emly did. It takes a lot to even begin questioning your beliefs, and it's exceptionally difficult for people who are deep in a conspiracy theory (such as those that drive the anti-vax movement), because for people in that position it's harder for evidence to break through. "Conspiracy theories are inherently self-sealing," write researchers Stephan Lewandowsky and John Cook in *The Conspiracy Theory Handbook.* "Evidence that counters a theory is re-interpreted as originating from the conspiracy."[49] For example, journalists and health professionals who call out wellness misinformation are often falsely accused of being in the pocket of "Big Pharma" or "Big Food" (as I may well be for writing this book). So the best way to challenge conspiracy theories isn't to debate and debunk, but rather to speak and listen empathetically, acknowledge the desire to think critically about the world, and help to redirect that critical-thinking energy to an analysis of the conspiracy theory itself.

An effective approach to dismantling conspiracy theories on a wider scale is to focus on the people who have *not* bought into them—the vast majority of people—and do what researchers call inoculation against misinformation, one technique of which is "prebunking": Give an explicit warning that there's an imminent threat of being misinformed, and then refute the arguments contained in the misinformation—without amplifying the misinformation itself. Prebunking alerts people to the kind of misinformation to watch out for and the manipulative techniques that may be used to get them to believe it. A 2022 study of nearly two thousand unvaccinated people found that prebunking helped them recognize and identify rhetorical strategies used in anti-vax content, reduced their likelihood of sharing that content, and made them more willing to get the COVID-19 vaccine.[50]

Another important way to dismantle anti-vax misinformation and other wellness conspiracy theories is to address the pernicious influence of social media. "Stated trust in social media is the biggest factor in the adoption of anti-vax attitudes," Imran Ahmed said in the 2021 webinar. Learning to have a robust skepticism of any health-related content you see on social media is one key to reducing your risk of falling into anti-vax conspiracies and other wellness traps. But social media companies also bear considerable blame for the mis- and disinformation on their platforms and should be held responsible for fixing the problem.

Amending Section 230 of the Communications Decency Act to make platforms liable for consequences stemming from the content they amplify would be a good way to do that. Although Section 230 reform has been stalled by political infighting thus far, a 2022 lawsuit showed a novel way that victims of social media misinformation might circumvent the law's limitations: The parents of a teenager named Alexis Spence, whom they allege was driven to a severe eating disorder by Instagram's algorithms, are suing parent company Meta for knowingly continuing to push pro-eating-disorder content to teens. As of this writing the suit is ongoing, and in it the parents are targeting Instagram's algorithms rather than its user-generated content (which is protected by Section 230), citing the Facebook Papers leaked by whistleblower Frances Haugen that show company executives knew its algorithm was harmful to teens' body image. As *Gizmodo* reported, "The lawsuit is among the first to use the documents against Meta in actual court rather than the court of public opinion."[51]

In the meantime, there are some steps social media users can take to help stem the spread of anti-vax propaganda and other mis- and disinformation.

For starters, while it can feel tempting to share this content in order to refute it, that's exactly what *not* to do. "The problem with misinformation is that all too often it triggers our desire to showcase it—to go, 'look at this absolute rubbish,'" Ahmed said—and yet sharing it just spreads the rubbish far and wide. Remember that social media algorithms are programmed to maximize engagement, and that content that provokes negative emotions like disgust and moral outrage tends to do that the best. Creators of mis- and disinformation use this feature (or flaw) of the algorithms to their benefit. So if we want to stop them, it's best to sit on our hands and *not* engage with the content, even when we feel an almost irresistible pull to respond. You might think of it as quarantining the misinformation in order to help reduce your own network's exposure to it. It's also counter-productive to argue with bots and trolls, because that helps them achieve their (or their programmers') goal of making it look like there's more debate about a given issue than there really is.

Another helpful guideline is to fact-check any source that evokes intense emotions in you, writes Marc-André Argentino, a researcher who studies how extremist groups manipulate tech platforms and algorithms to their advantage.[52] Of course it's under-standable and common to feel upset when reading about injustice—such as police violence or racially motivated attacks, for example—and you can verify these stories fairly easily by seeing if they're picked up by reputable news organizations that have a man-date to fact-check. (The efforts in recent years by right-wing politi-cians and bad actors to undermine the credibility of mainstream news outlets deliberately sows mistrust in these organizations, but they remain bound by laws and journalistic ethics that prohibit them from publishing falsehoods.) On the other hand, if a source provokes big feelings and you can't verify the facts, Argentino explains, there may be manipulation afoot. The source may be whipping up your emotions to try to sell you something…like an elderberry tincture or a $200 anti-vax docuseries. Or it might be trying to sow discord as a way of undermining democracy. Such is the case with disinformation actors like the Russian trolls and bots that spread both pro- and anti-vaccine content. Whatever you do, don't share a piece of information unless you've been able to verify it. "Each of us has remarkable power to amplify content," Renée DiResta writes. "That comes with a commensurate responsibility that most users haven't yet fully internalized."[53]

It also can be helpful to limit what you share online about your own health-related fears and hesitancies, especially when it comes to vaccines, given that the anti-vax industry specifically trains its workers to exploit fear. "They literally tell [their trainees], 'look for people expressing this fear,'" Ahmed said. "When someone says 'I'm just terrified,' that's the moment."

In some cases, however, a health scare can be the moment when people who are already in the anti-vax camp start reconsidering their views. It happened for Emly with the flu ordeal, which started her on a path that ultimately led her to get all her children (she now has three) up to date on their childhood immunizations, and to get them the COVID vaccine as soon as they were eligible. Simpson had a similar experience: In her anti-vax influencer heyday, when she was struggling with endometriosis and posted on Facebook about her decision to get surgery for the condition, the response from many people in her network was shocking. "All of my anti-vax friends were saying that I was taking the lazy route by having surgery, and that I just needed to eat better," Simpson told *Scary Mommy* in 2021. "I was so torn about that. I went to my gynecologist, and she hugged me, and she said, 'This isn't your fault.' And I cried and I cried because it was so relieving to hear that it wasn't my fault. The anti-vaxxers were saying if there was any health issue in your life, it's because of you."[54] Simpson says that experience with the doctor was the moment she started to turn toward Western medicine, and away from anti-vax views.

Personal-responsibility rhetoric and admonitions to "just eat better" are hallmarks of wellness culture, the outgrowth of an attitude and a practice that took root a half century or more ago. It is the belief—once a neoliberal talking point, then a battering ram, now endemic across the culture almost without regard to political persuasion—that physical health is the be-all and end-all of well-being, a goal that's attained primarily, if not entirely, through individual lifestyle choices.[55] Healthism, as this belief is called, doesn't align with the evidence on the importance of social determinants of health, but it's rampant in Western culture—in many corners of mainstream medicine, to be sure, but perhaps even more so in alternative and integrative spaces. In contrast, the acknowledgment by Simpson's doctor that her condition wasn't her fault, and the kindness and empathy that the provider conveyed, helped her start to understand that many, if not most, Western healthcare providers do care about their patients and aren't just callous shills for Big Pharma, as they're often made out to be in the anti-vax community.

Once Simpson started opening up to that possibility, she started looking with a newly critical eye at the anti-vax "facts" she'd previously found when she "did her research." One thing that really got her was the Vaccine Adverse Event Reporting System, or VAERS—the U.S. Department of Health and Human Services' portal for reporting issues with vaccines. Of course, a very small percentage of people genuinely do have serious reactions (or suspected serious reactions) to vaccines, which should be documented. But those reactions are only a fraction of what gets reported to VAERS. The database is publicly available and is full of truly wild and outlandish claims, which anti-vaxxers often use to argue that vaccines are dangerous. The unmoderated reports aren't scientific and definitely should not be used to establish that vaccines "caused" any of the outcomes described. Simpson started looking closely at the presumed adverse events listed and was shocked by what she saw: a gunshot wound, a fight in school, frostbite, an electric shock from a hair straightener, drowning, sunburn, STDs, sports injuries, suicidal ideation, murder, and many others. Thousands of people were claiming that vaccines were linked to totally unrelated things. "Anyone can report anything—with literally no proof," Simpson says.

The anti-vax position is an extreme one, to be sure. Certainly not everyone who gets involved with wellness culture will end up turning against vaccines, though social platforms have helped drive a disturbingly large number of people to take that turn. A more common path is to look to alternative or integrative medicine for help with unexplained symptoms and receive unproven diagnoses and so-called cures that in some cases make your problems far worse. It's these issues that we'll discuss next.

# CHAPTER 6

# Dubious Diagnoses and Spurious Cures

In 2012, Jody Esselstyn started suffering from a nebulous constellation of symptoms including fatigue, headaches, and joint pain. She went to her doctor, a Western-trained MD in a family practice, and got a diagnosis of Lyme disease. The doctor put her on an eight-week regimen of the antibiotic doxycycline—a slightly longer course than is usually recommended, since the doctor thought Esselstyn had probably had the infection for at least a few months. And it seemed to work; after the eight weeks, Esselstyn was back to feeling pretty good.

But then, not long afterwards, the fatigue and joint pain came back—and that's when the doctor started to deviate from conventional medicine. She started Esselstyn on a regimen that involved numerous (and costly) tinctures and herbal remedies, and kept her on it for months. "It's hard to say whether I felt better or not," says Esselstyn, a registered nurse. "I think I felt good about the fact that we were doing something to help me feel better, because I was just really desperate." In her early forties and with three young kids at home at the time, she felt like the fatigue was unsustainable.

She ultimately stayed on the herbal supplements for a year, at which point she decided to try going off them. Then she took a nursing job at a summer camp and came back feeling wiped out. Her doctor suspected that she had "adrenal fatigue"—an unsubstantiated diagnosis that's become popular in wellness culture. The claim is that constant stress causes the adrenal glands to become overtaxed and stop producing enough hormones. Esselstyn's doctor referred her to one of the nurse practitioners in her practice who specialized in functional medicine—a practice that purports to identify the root causes of illness (rather than simply managing symptoms) and generally uses diets as a first-line treatment.

Like so-called integrative medicine, functional medicine sits at the intersection of the conventional and alternative paradigms. Its practitioners are trained in the Western medical system and have recognized credentials—MD (medical doctor), NP (nurse practitioner)—but in addition to standard medical care they use some non-evidence-based methods that you'd be more likely to find in the office of a naturopath or chiropractor.

"I saw this NP and she said, yeah, for sure, based on your answers to this questionnaire about adrenal fatigue, you have it," Esselstyn says. Esselstyn had gained weight, and the NP pointed to that and long-standing fatigue as sure signs that she apparently had the condition. The NP also said it was possible that Esselstyn's Lyme disease might not have gone away, but she didn't push that; instead, she suggested first pursuing the "adrenal fatigue" diagnosis, which Esselstyn wanted to believe was correct. "It sounded cool, like maybe I can take the weight off and I can feel better, and it was all very appealing," she says.

The NP also told her that her hemoglobin A1C—a measure of average blood sugar over time—was borderline-high, right around the threshold of the "pre-diabetes" range. The provider recommended that Esselstyn take a steroid medication, which she said would help her energy levels and promote weight loss (though in fact steroid medications have actually been shown to *increase* the likelihood of high blood sugar and diabetes, as well as weight gain[1]). Although steroids may not seem very "natural," they're commonly used in functional medicine for so-called adrenal fatigue, supposedly to help jump-start the body's natural cortisol production. Even over-the-counter supplements for "adrenal support" often contain at least one steroid hormone, as well as thyroid hormone, a 2018 study found.[2] These drugs should be declared on the labels and administered only via prescription, but they're able to fly under the radar in the largely unregulated American supplement industry.

Soon Esselstyn was taking a passel of supplements, in addition to a low dose of a corticosteroid medication. This class of medication is known to help people feel better and more energetic at first, regardless of whether or not they need it. "Not surprisingly, I felt great," Esselstyn says. "I was on steroids." Perhaps because she was so excited to be feeling better, she didn't question whether steroids were really the right treatment—even though she knew, because of her training, that taking them was "actually kind of a bad idea." After a while, her blood-sugar readings weren't improving, so the NP prescribed a glucose monitor and instructed her to measure her blood sugar multiple times a day. Unfortunately, Esselstyn already had a very disordered relationship with food, and the constant blood-sugar monitoring fed right into it. "The eating-disorder brain was like, 'now I shouldn't eat that because of my blood sugar, and I should fast as much as possible.'"

As it happens, Esselstyn comes from something of a wellness-culture dynasty. Her uncle is Caldwell Esselstyn, a physician and author who claims that heart attacks can be entirely prevented by eating an austere, oil-free vegetarian diet.[3] One of her cousins—Caldwell's son, Rip Esselstyn (author of, among other titles, 2009's *The Engine 2 Diet* and *The Engine 2 Seven-Day Rescue Diet*, published in 2017)—is a former firefighter and triathlete and current plant-based diet entrepreneur who promotes the idea that "PLANTSTRONG" foods have the power to "protect, heal, and reverse disease."[4] Caldwell and Rip have been featured in numerous wellness documentaries including *Forks Over Knives*, *The Game Changers*, and *What the Health*—popular yet problematic films that advocate universal veganism for health reasons without sound evidence, and that have frightened many viewers into cutting out not just animal products but also, in some cases, all oils and most fats. Caldwell's wife and daughter, Ann and Jane Esselstyn, are also plant-based-diet evangelists and cookbook authors with a popular YouTube recipe channel. In the mid-1980s, when Caldwell first started advocating veganism for heart health, his younger brother—Jody's father— followed his lead and put his whole family on a strict vegan diet, including then-fifteen-year-old Jody. For her, a perfectionistic teenager, this restriction—combined with her family's overall rhetoric around food—helped spark a decades-long struggle with disordered eating.

"One of their phrases is 'moderation equals death,' " she says of her uncle and aunt. "So you're either all in, or you're not doing it right and you're going to die of heart disease." To be fair, she says, her uncle works with the most serious heart-disease patients—many of whom have such advanced cases that they aren't even eligible for open-heart surgery—and she believes he has made a difference for a lot of these patients. "But I think the collateral damage is so great for people like me or other folks who are like, 'maybe I'll go plant based for the planet,' but then find themselves in this rabbit hole where there's so much demonizing of processed food," she says. Around the time her family went vegan, her aunt and uncle asked her what her favorite food was. She said peanut butter, thinking that was a good answer because it's vegan. "My uncle said, 'Oh, it's pure lard,' " she remembers. "He was so fatphobic, but that just stuck with me. I'm fifty and I still remember that moment."

For someone with a history like Esselstyn's, how do you tease apart the symptoms of an eating disorder from the symptoms of another condition? And how do you know which of the conditions you've been diagnosed with—like "adrenal fatigue" or other wellness-culture labels—even exist?

Constellations of nebulous symptoms—like the fatigue, joint pain, and headaches that Esselstyn suffered, as well as others like brain fog, depression, and digestive issues—are all too real for millions of people, especially women. And yet conventional medicine often struggles to provide satisfactory diagnoses, let alone treatments, for these conditions—particularly when it comes to post-infectious syndromes like post-treatment Lyme disease syndrome (often referred to by patients as "chronic Lyme") or post-acute COVID-19 syndrome (aka long COVID). These issues are "at the edge of medical knowledge," writes Meghan O'Rourke in her 2022 book on chronic illness, *The Invisible Kingdom.*[5] Living at that edge can be incredibly painful, and trying to find answers and satisfactory treatments can swallow years or even decades of your life. Understandably, some people become so desperate in those situations that they'll try anything.

The feeling that conventional medicine doesn't have an answer for you, coupled with the fact that some doctors treat chronically ill patients as if it's "all in their head," has created a void that dubious diagnoses and spurious cures come to fill. Conspiracy theories involving Big Pharma and the medical-industrial complex help drive many of these diagnoses, including adrenal fatigue, chronic candida, and leaky gut syndrome, among others. Many of these labels derive from grains of truth about the human body, intermingled with misinformation and distorted by a wellness industry that capitalizes on people's pain.

Of course not all wellness practitioners are fonts of misinformation, and most aren't maliciously trying to prey on vulnerable patients. Many of them go into their fields with a genuine desire to help people. Moreover, there's no shortage of people (maybe even you or others you know) who believe that their naturopath, functional-medicine doctor, chiropractor, or other integrative- or alternative-medicine provider changed their lives for the better. About half of Americans report having tried some form of alternative medicine during their lifetime, according to a 2017 Pew Research Center report: about 20 percent have used it instead of conventional medicine, whereas about 30 percent say they've used it in conjunction with standard medical treatment.[6] That's a lot of people, and undoubtedly some of them were very happy with their treatments. I don't pretend to have all the answers, and it's certainly possible that some of the wellness-culture practices I'm criticizing really do work for some people some of the time.

But there are also many reasons why those practices might *seem* to work that have little to do with the practices themselves. One reason could be that a practitioner finally gave you the empathy and support that you needed—and that we all deserve from our healthcare providers—which has been shown to help improve well-being. For example, a randomized controlled trial of more than 250 people with irritable bowel syndrome found that patients who received acupuncture treatment from a warm, empathetic, and attentive provider had a significant reduction in symptoms—equivalent to the effects of a powerful IBS drug—compared to patients who received the treatment from a brusque provider who didn't spend time talking with them.[7] In fact, both of the supposed treatments used "sham" acupuncture needles that didn't pierce the skin, so the effects didn't have anything to do with acupuncture itself, but rather with the ritual of the "treatment" and the relationship between practitioner and patient. Integrative- and alternative-medicine practitioners typically are able to give a lot more time and attention to each patient than conventional doctors (in some cases because the former don't take insurance and instead command high out-of-pocket fees), and that goes a long way toward helping people feel better. The claim that they "treat the whole person" isn't always borne out, because often they're just prescribing diets and treating physical health, as we'll discuss. But to the extent that they offer empathy and time, alternative-medicine providers may help address mental health, too, in a way that the Western medical system—with its insurance plans and brisk 15-minute appointments—just isn't set up to do.

The power of empathy from care providers is one of several *placebo effects* that can explain the benefits seen in many alternative and integrative treatments. You've likely heard of the singular "placebo effect" (where someone takes an inert sugar pill and feels better because they believed it was a real drug), but researchers who study this concept are starting to view it more as a plural noun. "I see the placebo effect as a kind of loose family of different phenomena that are just yoked together by this term," Franklin Miller, a retired NIH bioethicist who has edited a book on the placebo effect, told *Vox* in 2017.[8] Placebo effects include all the various ways that the mind can help to create genuine healing for the body, such as the "care effect" discussed above, and the phenomenon whereby many people will get better results from a treatment when they observe that *other* people feel better when taking it (even if the treatment itself is inert).[9]

Far from being "all in our heads," placebo effects can produce real clinical results for conditions that come with a direct mind-body connection—things like pain, nausea, and phobias. In those situations, the rituals involved in placebo treatments can potentially have a genuine impact on symptoms (though some people are more responsive to placebo effects than others). But the placebo effect doesn't work for conditions like cancer, because as much as some wellness influencers claim that cancer is a manifestation of "toxic" thoughts, it's actually caused by cancerous cells—and our minds can't direct our bodies to kill those cells, no matter how hard we try. Placebo effects can help treat symptoms, but they don't address the root cause of disease (which is ironic, given that wellness culture constantly says the same about Western medicine).

A close cousin of placebo effects is what's known as the nocebo effect—when the mere belief that something is harmful causes you to experience genuine pain and other symptoms. The nocebo effect often takes hold when someone has negative expectations of, or has had previous bad experiences with, a certain treatment or medication, be it pharmaceuticals or gluten. In fact, the nocebo effect is common among people who believe that they have non-celiac gluten sensitivity. Because gluten is demonized in diet and wellness culture, it has become easy to conclude that you might be sensitive to it. On the other side of the equation, there are researchers who believe that this condition may not exist at all (even though the symptoms may be very real), as I discussed in *Anti-Diet.*[10]

Another reason wellness-culture treatments might seem to work is a phenomenon known as regression to the mean. The concept comes from statistics, and it shows that extreme outcomes typically become less extreme—moving toward the average or mean—over time. In medicine, regression to the mean happens with symptoms: most illnesses will get better with time, so if enough time goes by you're likely to end up feeling better, no matter what wellness-culture practices you do (or don't) engage in. People often seek treatment or enroll in clinical trials when their symptoms become unbearable or are at their worst, so regression to the mean is often inevitable—and it can even make it look like placebos are having more of an effect than they really are.[11] Indeed, many chronic diseases involve normal symptom fluctuations, and sometimes symptoms will happen to ebb right after a certain treatment, in a way that makes it seem as if the treatment is effective, when really it is not.

In fact, a substantial amount of scientific research into many popular alternative-medicine treatments has shown little to no evidence of effectiveness. Despite the common refrain that there's no funding for research on so-called integrative medicine, there's actually quite a bit: between 1999 and 2019 (the last year for which data was available as of this writing), the National Institutes of Health spent more than $6.6 billion on that research.[12] (The NIH budget comes from taxpayers, so many of us are actually helping finance alternative-medicine studies, though the bulk of that budget still goes to studying conventional medicine.) In 2019 alone, the NIH spent $517.2 million on research into complementary and alternative medicine—a good 2,600 times more, in inflation-adjusted dollars, than when government funding for this research first began. The old adage that there was no money to study alternative therapies may have been true back then, but two-plus decades later the reality is very different.

And most of this research has been disappointing for proponents of wellness culture. Over the years the federal government has spent $750,000 to find that prayer doesn't cure AIDS or reduce recovery time for breast-reconstruction surgery; $700,000 to find that magnets don't help with arthritis, migraines, or carpal tunnel syndrome; $406,000 to find that coffee enemas don't cure pancreatic cancer; and millions of dollars for other null results.[13] NIH-funded research has found that a very small number of complementary- and alternative-medicine treatments may be effective for certain conditions, such as ginger for chemotherapy nausea or yoga and meditation for anxiety, but overall the results of these trials have not shown benefits for most alternative therapies. The conspiracist take on this might be that the studies were done by biased researchers, but in fact the NIH often gives money directly to alternative-medicine providers to set up and run the trials themselves—including millions of dollars in grants to naturopathic institutions such as the Bastyr University Research Institute and the National University of Natural Medicine.[14]

So if you're someone who feels you were helped by wellness-culture practices, I'm genuinely happy for you and would never want to detract from your healing. At the same time, if you're open to it, I'd invite you to consider that perhaps what made the difference in your symptoms wasn't necessarily (or entirely) the particular wellness treatment you engaged in, but some of these other factors instead. The wellness industry is quick to take credit for any improvements in people's well-being—and to harness social media algorithms to spread that message—when in fact it's often your body's natural healing process, your relationship with an empathetic care provider, or some other aspect of the mind-body connection that truly deserves the recognition.

When wellness culture hogs the glory in this way, the stories that often go untold are the ones where patients were *not* helped— or in some cases were deeply harmed—by alternative-medicine approaches. People often simply move on to other providers when this happens and may not talk about their bad experiences, or they may not connect it to alternative/integrative/functional medicine in particular (since so many of us have had bad experiences in the conventional medical system, too). But once you start digging into some of the most common wellness-culture diagnoses and treatments, it becomes clear just how problematic they really are. These dubious diagnoses and spurious cures often trigger and exacerbate disordered eating. They also can distract from the true causes of certain symptoms, causing people to waste precious time and money on ineffective and harmful regimens instead of getting the help they deserve. The consequences of delaying treatment or of seeking ineffective cures can be deadly. And when people start believing in false disease labels, it can expose them to increasing levels of mis- and disinformation. As this cycle perpetuates, the wellness industry takes advantage of people who are desperate and vulnerable to false promises of relief. Even well-meaning providers may unwittingly do so.

### Adrenal Fatigue

When she was pregnant with her third child, Christina (a pseudonym) suffered from extreme nausea and vomiting. None of the tricks she'd used in previous pregnancies were working: frequent meals, ginger, over-the-counter and prescription medications recommended by her doctor. "I was doing everything I could think of to help with it," she says. "I'm a dietitian and I was working at an eating-disorder center, and it's really hard to be struggling with nausea and vomiting when you're trying to run cooking groups and trying to eat. I just wanted relief." Desperate and willing to try things she hadn't considered before, she decided to follow a family member's recommendation and went to a local chiropractor for acupuncture.

When she went in for her appointment, though, not only did she find no relief from the acupuncture, but she also got a surprising diagnosis: adrenal fatigue. The chiropractor didn't do any tests; like Esselstyn's NP, he based his opinion on a questionnaire that Christina had filled out with her new-client forms. The questions asked her to rate things like her sleep quality, stress level, energy levels — all of which can be impacted by pregnancy *itself* and don't necessarily mean anything is amiss. But to the chiropractor, they were apparently enough to warrant a diagnosis. "Looking back, how could he make such a claim on just a few questions on a questionnaire?" Christina says. "There wasn't any looking into my body or asking additional questions. It was just diagnosed so easily: 'this is adrenal fatigue, and this is how you should fix it... this supplement will cure it.'"

That was her first clue that something about this supposed diagnosis wasn't right.

The adrenal glands are small, triangle-shaped organs that sit on top of each kidney and produce hormones that help regulate the body's metabolism, immune system, blood pressure, stress response, and more. The term "adrenal fatigue" was coined in 1998 by a naturopath and chiropractor named James Wilson, who subsequently wrote a 2001 book outlining the supposed diagnosis and his method of treatment. On page 61 of the book is a questionnaire developed and used by Wilson to identify the condition.[15] Wilson's theory, which is unsupported by scientific evidence, is that the adrenal glands get overworked by excessive stress and stop making enough of the hormones our bodies need, particularly cortisol.[16] His book was published by a small press that specializes in alternative health and might never have reached a wide audience, but the explosion of wellness culture over the past twenty years has probably helped increase the book's popularity, to the point where two websites selling supplements under Wilson's name have claimed that the book has sold more than 800,000 copies—a major success by publishing-industry standards.[17] Today, many integrative- and alternative-medicine practitioners use the questionnaire from Wilson's book (or some variation on it, like the intake questions used by Christina's chiropractor) to "diagnose" adrenal fatigue.

The problem is that adrenal fatigue isn't a real condition.

The symptoms people experience are very real, of course. Far too many of us feel exhausted all the time without knowing why, and conventional medicine often doesn't have great answers. "I just felt really run down and really not vital, like I'd been hit by a truck," said Erin Todd, another woman who was misdiagnosed as having adrenal fatigue. "I had no energy and no desire. Clearly something was wrong." But the diagnosis itself is a dubious one, considered false by experts on hormonal conditions. "Adrenal fatigue is not an actual disease," said Anat Ben-Shlomo, an endocrinologist at the Cedars-Sinai Adrenal Program, in a 2018 interview.[18] "Stress can have an impact on our health, but it doesn't affect your adrenals this way. When you're stressed, the adrenal glands actually produce more of the cortisol and other hormones you need. They will give you all that's necessary."

A 2016 review of the scientific literature, published in a reputable journal of endocrine disorders, had a title that was notably frank for a scientific study: "Adrenal Fatigue Does Not Exist: A Systematic Review."[19] It looked at the results of fifty-eight studies with more than 12,000 total participants spanning two decades and found that none of the studies supported the concept of adrenal fatigue; none of them even used appropriate methods to test whether there was any correlation between participant-reported fatigue and adrenal function. The Endocrine Society, a group of physicians and researchers specializing in hormone health, has been sounding the alarm on this dubious diagnosis for years. "No scientific proof exists to support adrenal fatigue as a true medical condition," the group wrote in 2022. "Doctors urge you not to waste precious time accepting an unproven diagnosis such as adrenal fatigue if you feel tired, weak, or depressed."[20]

Even James Wilson, the author who came up with the concept of so-called adrenal fatigue, seems to acknowledge that there's no real scientific evidence behind it. As the official version of his questionnaire cautions, "No formal reliability or validity tests have been completed to confirm its accuracy, and the author assumes no responsibility for its use or accuracy."[21]

Proponents of adrenal fatigue will say that Western medicine is simply ignoring alternative evidence so that it can continue to profit off people's ongoing symptoms. But if anyone is profiting in this case, it would seem to be the practitioners who diagnose adrenal fatigue, and the wellness entrepreneurs who sell the purported cures (who are sometimes one and the same). People diagnosed with the supposed disease report taking dozens of supplements to treat it, spending thousands of dollars on out-of-pocket expenses, since insurance generally won't cover unproven diseases. Treatments recommended for adrenal fatigue range from supplements that are probably benign, if ineffective and expensive, to more dangerous interventions.

In particular, there's treatment with corticosteroids, synthetic versions of the cortisol produced naturally by the adrenal glands, like Esselstyn's NP prescribed. Practitioners who recommend corticosteroids to patients for supposed adrenal fatigue claim that patients' own cortisol levels are depleted, pointing to the immediate and significant improvements these patients tend to experience on corticosteroids.[22] Yet that's not necessarily evidence that the medications are needed. As Esselstyn noted, corticosteroids are known to create a temporary boost in people's sense of well-being regardless of their condition. What's more, even at low doses mirroring the hormone levels that would normally be found in the body, corticosteroids have been found to increase the risk of a number of health problems, including osteoporosis, glaucoma, sleep disturbances, cardiovascular disease, and metabolic, muscular, and psychiatric disorders.[23] The Endocrine Society cautions that supplements used to treat so-called adrenal fatigue may not be safe: "If you take adrenal hormone supplements when you don't need them, your adrenal glands may stop working and become unable to make the hormones you need when you are under physical stress. When these supplements are stopped, a person's adrenal glands can remain 'asleep' for months. People with this problem may be in danger of developing a life-threatening condition called adrenal crisis."[24]

Christina's chiropractor, for example, recommended that she take adrenal extract from pigs. "I said no thanks, as that didn't seem safe, especially being pregnant," she says. She knew enough about supplements to know that the pills probably weren't tested for safety or efficacy because the industry is so loosely regulated. She ended up deciding to forgo the risky treatment and just suffer through the nausea and vomiting for several more weeks. "I luckily wasn't so desperate that I would be willing to try it," she says. But unfortunately, many others are desperate enough to try just about anything.

Although so-called adrenal fatigue isn't real, there is a true condition that *sounds* similar: adrenal insufficiency, a rare disorder in which the adrenal glands don't produce enough of the hormones they should, including cortisol and aldosterone. The difference is that adrenal insufficiency doesn't happen because you've "overtaxed your adrenals," but rather because of legitimate physical or environmental causes: In primary adrenal insufficiency, also known as Addison's disease (which is the rarer type of adrenal insufficiency), the adrenal glands are damaged by an autoimmune response, impairing their ability to secrete hormones. In secondary adrenal insufficiency, a problem with the pituitary gland can cause it to produce too little adrenocorticotropic hormone (ACTH), which normally stimulates the adrenal glands to produce cortisol. Or, more frequently, *taking corticosteroid medications* can also cause secondary adrenal insufficiency, because the body reduces or shuts down its own production of cortisol in response to the medication. In fact, long-term use of these steroids is the most common cause of adrenal insufficiency.[25] That means one of the very things that integrative and functional-medicine providers use to treat people for the nonexistent disease of "adrenal fatigue" can actually *cause* people to develop a very real disorder of the adrenal glands.

What's more, the false diagnosis of adrenal fatigue can keep people from getting the help they need for true medical conditions—whether they have adrenal insufficiency or something else. For Esselstyn, the true cause of the fatigue and joint pain that initially brought her to the functional-medicine NP could potentially have been the lingering effects of Lyme disease, even after the disease was long gone, though she never did hear that from her doctors. She now thinks the fatigue also could have been related to anemia, as well as to the exhausting juggle of work and kids. And it may have had something to do with her eating disorder, which was finally diagnosed as anorexia in 2020 after years of flying under the radar.

For Todd as well, the real issue was likely in how she was relating to food and her body. "I don't think anything was ever wrong with my adrenals," she says. Instead, she believes she probably had an undiagnosed eating disorder, which can cause all the same symptoms as supposed adrenal fatigue, including exhaustion and gastrointestinal issues—particularly constipation. Looking back, Todd sees clearly how her restrictive eating was at play. "I wasn't eating enough to produce a bowel movement," she says. And once she started eating more and stopped restricting all the foods that had been off limits on her "clean" diet, those issues essentially vanished. She went from having severe symptoms after eating particular foods while on a juice cleanse, to being totally fine with those foods after coming off it.

For Christina, the false diagnosis of adrenal fatigue masked a happier explanation: she was pregnant with twins. (Multiple births generally produce more hormones, which may cause more nausea.) She was lucky in that she never got dangerously dehydrated from the vomiting, and her symptoms improved significantly in the second trimester, which they often do. She never returned to that chiropractor.

### *Leaky Gut Syndrome*

I interviewed another woman named Erin, who asked that only her first name be used. This Erin has struggled with psoriasis for her entire adult life. Now in her early forties, she's softspoken and has a youthful energy. She lives in northern Alberta, Canada, about five hours from the nearest major city, so she wasn't able to find many options for treating psoriasis other than going the pharmaceutical route. Her doctor recommended a topical steroid, which she didn't think seemed like a good long-term solution, both because she has melanoma in the family and is at higher risk for skin cancer (for which long-term use of topical steroids may raise the risk, though a 2018 systematic review found no evidence to establish whether or not this is true),[26] and because eventually steroid treatments stopped working well to control her condition. She also felt uneasy about taking biologics—systemic medications that suppress the part of the immune system that's overactive in psoriasis—and unfortunately none of her doctors took the time to talk her through these options. "I've had so many poor experiences with medical doctors who sort of shame or just don't have the time for you, or certainly haven't met me in my hesitation," she says. "I always seem to get the doctor who's like, 'just trust me,'" but that never sat well with her.

So it was no surprise that she was attracted to alternative medicine. "It really appealed to me to be like, okay, I'm in control here," she says. In addition to the psoriasis, she was also suffering from migraines and severe chronic stomach pain, as well as struggling with anxiety, depression, and exhaustion. She'd never gotten good support for those things, so when she heard about the naturopathic approach, it immediately resonated. It felt like finally she was going to have someone listen to her, take her symptoms seriously, and figure out what was going on. And when she started working with a naturopathic doctor, she got a diagnosis that supposedly explained the cause of all these disparate problems: "leaky gut syndrome."

That diagnosis, unfortunately, is another dubious one. Providers who diagnose so-called leaky gut syndrome claim that it's a condition that causes bacteria and toxins to "leak" through holes in the intestinal wall, in turn provoking other problems: digestive, psychological, autoimmune (including skin disorders like psoriasis). Scientific evidence doesn't support this hypothesis, but the supposed syndrome is based on a few kernels of truth: first, our intestines are selectively permeable, which allows water and nutrients to be absorbed into our bloodstream. If we didn't have some degree of intestinal permeability, we wouldn't be able to extract essential nutrients from our food. So "intestinal permeability" is real, but it's perfectly normal. The second grain of truth in the "leaky gut syndrome" story is that there's a genuine thing called *increased* intestinal permeability (aka intestinal hyperpermeability), which is when the intestine becomes more permeable than it would otherwise be. (Confusingly, some researchers and medical doctors refer to increased intestinal permeability in lay terms as "leaky gut," even when they're not talking about the hypothetical "leaky gut syndrome" or diagnosing anyone with the supposed condition.) Increased intestinal permeability has been found in some people who have gastrointestinal disorders such as celiac disease, Crohn's disease, and irritable bowel syndrome, and may also be associated with some other conditions. The science on this is still in its infancy, but the research so far only shows that increased intestinal permeability is *correlated* with those diseases—not the *cause* of the diseases or their symptoms, as many people in wellness culture argue. (Remember the golden rule in statistics: correlation does not equal causation.) In fact, researchers generally view increased intestinal permeability as a symptom of these conditions, not a cause.

Because there's no scientific evidence that increased intestinal permeability causes any disease or symptoms, the so-called leaky gut syndrome that providers like Erin's naturopath diagnose isn't a recognized medical condition, and there are no validated tests for it. Scientists are currently debating the validity of different tests to use in further *research* on intestinal permeability—which, again, is in the early stages and is primarily being conducted on animals, not in large-scale trials of humans. Given the state of the science, at-home tests or lab tests offered in healthcare providers' offices claiming to diagnose "leaky gut" should be viewed with extreme skepticism (though I know how powerful it is to think you've finally found the explanation for symptoms you've been struggling with for years without relief).

Similarly, treatments for this so-called syndrome are speculative at best. Most of them are just standard wellness-diet fare:

obsessively cut out the foods deemed "bad" in diet and wellness culture, and replace them with "whole" foods and supplements. These are essentially the same prescriptions that many alternative- and integrative-medicine providers offer for a litany of other con- ditions, without solid science to back them up.

That doesn't stop many such providers from ordering tests and prescribing treatments for this supposed disorder. Erin says her naturopathic doctor quickly diagnosed her with "leaky gut syndrome" after advising her to undergo "food intolerance" testing—which is often misleading and harmful, as we dis- cussed in Chapter 1. "I had to eliminate a tremendous amount of food, and what I was still allowed to eat had to be 'clean,'" she says.

Unsurprisingly, her relationship with food became very dis- ordered in this process, as it does for many people with this sup- posed diagnosis. "I joke that during this time I was limited to organic lettuce and plain brown rice cakes, but that's not far from the truth," she says. The ND told her she was intolerant of sugar, dairy, vegetables and fruits from the nightshade family, and many other foods. She started to see food as dangerous. Looking back now, she recognizes that that's when she devel- oped orthorexia—a type of disordered eating characterized by an obsession with the healthfulness and "purity" of foods. She also was overexercising and training for triathlons, and her rela- tionship with physical activity became very disordered as well, as is common for many people with orthorexia. She cut out sugar completely for a few years, to the point where she was even mak- ing her own ketchup from scratch. "It was such a burden because I felt then that it was up to me to heal myself," she says of that time in her life. "I was also on a long, expensive, and overwhelm- ing cocktail of supplements, homeopathics, ointments, shakes, and tinctures, in addition to the burden of a limited diet." At one point, she was taking at least twenty different supplements a day, stored in two big pillboxes that were filled to overflowing.

Not only did she develop an eating disorder, but her psoriasis didn't improve at all; in fact, it got worse. But at the time Erin didn't see the connection between the naturopath's recommendations and her declining condition, in large part because of the provider's refrain—a common one among wellness-culture practitioners—that things would get worse before they got better, and that feeling bad means the treatment is "working." Erin went off the steroid medication, and sure enough, her psoriasis flared up. "I saw it worsen right away," she says, but she thought that was a sign that "toxins" were coming out as part of the process of healing her leaky gut. She acknowledges that she probably was experiencing some sunk-cost bias as well, having invested so much time and money in the naturopathic approach that she didn't want to give up before seeing the promised benefits that were supposedly just around the corner. But those benefits never came. "I think within a year or so, it got to the point where my whole torso was covered [with lesions] and I couldn't even put on a shirt without my skin just, like, separating," she says. "It was worse right away and sustained throughout—I don't think I really ever had any relief."

Adding insult to injury, the treatment was incredibly expensive. Between the special tests she had to pay for out of pocket, the supplements, and the appointments themselves, she spent more than $5,000 (CAN) over the course of eight years working with this naturopath. Healthcare is generally free in Canada, but neither the public health plan nor her husband's private insurance would cover the naturopathic doctor because they don't see this form of treatment as evidence-based.

After Erin had spent years working with this ND, who she really believes was trying her best to help, it became clear that the efforts at healing her "leaky gut syndrome" weren't working—at which point, the ND "began to throw things at me to see what would stick." There was talk of metal toxicity, then adrenal fatigue. It all started to seem like a big guessing game, and for Erin that was the tipping point. She stopped seeing the naturopath and tried to make a go of it on her own.

She sometimes gets down on herself about having gone so far down the alternative-medicine path, but the fact that she was willing to pay so much for—and devote so many years of her life to—this treatment that ultimately failed says a lot about how desperate she was for answers, and how much she wanted it to work. She also feels that if she hadn't tried the naturopathic approach, part of her would still be wondering if it was actually the key to healing for her. As someone with multiple chronic conditions that it took years to get properly diagnosed and treated, I can very much empathize with that position. When you believe you've finally found an explanation and a solution for your symptoms, it feels like an enormous burden has been lifted and you can breathe again. Having to come to terms with the fact that the diagnosis and treatment were incorrect feels like having to voluntarily re-shoulder that burden and trudge on into unknown territory. It's hard to do that until you're really certain it's not going to work.

Of course, not all naturopaths (or alternative practitioners of other persuasions) would have continued to pursue a treatment regimen for that long when it obviously wasn't working. But Erin's experience—the fact that this provider stuck to one explanation, "leaky gut," for years, in the absence of any clear evidence of its correctness—is unfortunately far too common. Many of the people I've spoken with about wellness-culture approaches to chronic illness went through the same thing. Often it seems that even the most well-intentioned provider will have a favorite explanation for what's ailing every one of their patients—whether it's food intolerance, overworked adrenal glands, leaky intestines, or something else—and they'll support it with a flawed test (or questionnaire) that's pretty much guaranteed to produce the results they're looking for.

This kind of thing has been going on for years in the

complementary- and alternative-medicine field—sometimes in good faith, and sometimes not. In 1990, *Inside Edition* aired an exposé about a "diet doctor" in New York City who gave two patients (one a reporter, the other a prominent allergist) the same diagnosis of chronic fatigue syndrome and candida, after spending about two minutes with each of them and doing no physical examination.[27] One of his former employees said the doctor had instructed his staff to indicate on blood-test reports that *every* patient who came through their doors was allergic to wheat, dairy products, eggs, and yeast.

Although the wellness industry talks a big game about "treating the whole person" and not giving one-size-fits-all solutions, alternative and integrative providers can be surprisingly wedded to their pet theories, and in the process can fail to truly listen to their patients or treat them as unique individuals. Instead they give the same set of answers to everyone, even when those clearly don't meet the needs of a given patient, and in that sense they can be just as dismissive as the Western medicine they're so apt to criticize. Erin believes that's what happened with her ND—"leaky gut" was the default hypothesis, which the provider confirmed with a dubious test and then treated by eliminating foods. Today, now that Erin has come to recognize this pattern, she sees it all over the wellness world. One glaring example is the Medical Medium, the uncredentialed influencer we discussed in Chapter 1: "He's like, hmm, yes, I hear your problems, and you know what the answer is? The thing that I always default to: celery juice."

### Chronic Candida

Before Kristin (who asked that only her first name be used) started seeing her allergist as a patient in 2010, she'd known her socially for many years through the church they both attended.

They'd had numerous positive interactions in that time, and the allergist had a great reputation in their small city. She was a Western-trained MD who'd gone to the local medical school that several of Kristin's friends had also attended, but she also had a bit of a holistic vibe that Kristin liked.

One day Kristin took her daughter to youth camp and ran into the allergist, who was working that weekend as a camp nurse. They got to talking, and Kristin confided that she'd recently had surgery and was having a hard time recovering from it. She was constantly fatigued, and in fact had been for many years, but she'd had a hard time finding help from conventional medical doctors. In college, one had told her that she was just depressed and needed antidepressants. Later, another doctor told her that she was tired all the time because she had kids. She had been diagnosed with IBS when she was eighteen, and the doctor she saw for that told her the digestive problems were caused by "emotional issues." Like many people with chronic conditions who are told it's all in their head, she felt the medical system had failed her, so she was seeking out a nontraditional approach.

When she told the allergist about her symptoms at camp that day, the doctor didn't examine her or run any tests, but she said she thought it was likely an overgrowth of yeast—specifically candida—and recommended that Kristin come and see her. But because the doctor had a long waiting list, she recommended that while waiting for an appointment Kristin read a book about all the supposed conditions caused by candida. "I remember reading that book and just being kind of floored because they were listing out a lot of the things that I had been dealing with for years and years and years, because it wasn't just the fatigue," she says. "There was a laundry list of symptoms, from serious headaches to acne to constant GI distress to insomnia." Kristin had been trying to get help for these issues since she was a teenager, and it seemed that here, at last, was the answer.

At their first appointment, the doctor tested for a slew of environmental allergies—typical airborne things like different pollens, dust mites, and mold. "I [tested] positive [for] everything except for corn smut, whatever that is," Kristin says. The doctor started her on allergy drops and shots right away, which she says was life-changing. Previously she would get sick twice a year with what she thought was a bad cold that inevitably turned into bronchitis and lasted up to six weeks, but after the allergy testing she realized that these seemingly viral illnesses were actually an extreme case of hay fever from the pollens in the air at those times of year. The allergy drops and shots—mainstays in the medical treatment of allergies, with substantial scientific evidence behind them—made a world of difference.

Because that part of the process worked so well, Kristin felt she had no reason to question the other advice the doctor gave her. Even though the allergy tests they had done hadn't included yeast, the doctor diagnosed Kristin with candida based on her medical history alone. The allergist then prescribed "a hyper-restrictive diet that makes most people cry when they actually see it," Kristin says. The testing the doctor had done for environmental allergies had already proven to be tremendously helpful, so Kristin had no reason to disbelieve the candida diagnosis. She did have an environmental allergy to mold, after all, so the idea that yeast was a problem didn't seem so far-fetched. It was also just a huge relief to find a provider who seemed to have real answers. "She was really the first person to say, 'we can fix this, I know exactly what's wrong with you,'" Kristin says.

Over the past several decades, many people like Kristin have been told that they have issues with yeast—organisms that are members of the kingdom Fungi, which also includes mushrooms, mold, mildew, and a few other fungal species that cause plant diseases (including, as it happens, corn smut). Alternative- and integrative-medicine providers who diagnose candida often claim that the yeast is overgrowing throughout most people's bodies, causing disparate, chronic symptoms, despite no scientific evidence to support that theory. It's true that candida can overgrow in parts of the body for certain people under specific circumstances, but the concept of "candida overgrowth" as packaged and sold by wellness culture is largely pseudoscience—and the idea that people with this supposed condition can go on restrictive diets to "starve the yeast" is not evidence based.

Candida is a fungus that naturally lives in and on our bodies, and it's a constituent of the microbiome that the wellness world is so obsessed with these days. Because it's ubiquitous, candida can sometimes overgrow in specific locations under certain circumstances, just like other organisms in our microbiome. Probably the most common example of this is a vaginal yeast infection (*Candida* vulvovaginitis, or vulvovaginal candidiasis), which most people with vaginas have experienced at least once, and around half have had repeatedly.[28] It's also possible to get yeast infections in the mouth (oral thrush), skin folds, navel, penis, anus, and nail beds. Risk factors for these types of candida infections include long-term use of antibiotics or steroid medications, the use of oral contraceptives or IUDs, pregnancy, poorly controlled diabetes, rare genetic immune disorders, and other immunocompromised states (more on those shortly).

Dietary interventions have not been proven to help treat or prevent these garden-variety yeast infections, but numerous non-diet interventions have. If possible, getting off any medications that may be contributing to vaginal yeast infections—like oral contraceptives or IUDs—is often helpful. Using topical and/or intravaginal antifungal creams is another evidence-based method for treating these infections (and stopping the itching they cause), as are oral antifungal medications for more severe cases.[29] Probiotics also have been studied with mixed results, with some studies indicating they may offer some short-term help in treating vaginal yeast infections, while others have found that probiotics don't seem to help with treatment or prevention.[30]

It's also technically true that people can have candida infections throughout their bodies, but not in the way that wellness culture claims. A small percentage of the population is susceptible to a very real and serious condition called systemic candidiasis (invasive candidiasis), which couldn't be more different from the "systemic candida" that alternative and integrative providers like Kristin's allergist diagnose. (I also just want to point out that finding the right language to distinguish between true and false conceptions of candida can be difficult because of how wellness culture has co-opted and twisted medical terminology to serve its own pseudoscientific ends, which is why I'm using quotation marks here to signify when I'm talking about the ersatz condition as opposed to a real one.) *True* systemic candidiasis is a life-threatening fungal infection of the bloodstream, causing symptoms including low blood pressure, fast heart rate, rapid breathing, and fever and chills that don't improve with antibiotics.[31] Invasive candidiasis can also affect other bodily systems, including the brain and spinal cord, abdomen, heart, kidneys, liver, bones, muscles, joints, spleen, and/or eyes, causing various symptoms depending on the part of the body that's infected. But—and this is incredibly important—invasive candidiasis only affects a very small percentage of people, at most about two hundredths of a percent of the population.[32] Sufferers typically have specific, serious risk factors: HIV/AIDS, severe immunodeficiency, hematologic cancers, previous undiagnosed bloodstream infections, and so on; or they were hospitalized long-term, had a central IV line, or were on long-term antibiotics, for instance.

Unfortunately, over the past several decades, wellness culture has been spreading the false beliefs that "systemic candida" is a chronic condition, not an acute one, and that it can happen to anyone. It all started with two doctors in the 1970s and '80s who blamed candida for pretty much all unexplained illness; then, the explosion of wellness culture in subsequent decades helped disseminate their message far and wide. Today, many wellness providers, influencers, and websites falsely claim that "candida overgrowth" causes a laundry list of symptoms that are both wildly disparate and incredibly common—these include acne, allergies, asthma, autoimmune diseases, bloating, body odor, brain fog, constipation, dizziness, fatigue, food cravings, headaches, impotence, insomnia, joint pain, low sex drive, mood swings, rashes, thinning hair, and weight gain. "Candida overgrowth" (aka "chronic candida," "candidiasis hypersensitivity syndrome," "yeast syndrome," or "yeast overgrowth") has become a popular diagnosis in certain wellness circles likely because it *seems* to account for so many otherwise unexplained ailments from which people understandably are seeking relief. The recommended "treatments" for the supposed condition include an austere diet that restricts sugar, carbs, yeast, and some other foods, on the belief that these "feed" the candida. Other prescriptions include probiotics, bone-broth "cleanses," and of course scores and scores of supplements. Some patients are also put on multiple courses of oral antifungal medications, often without any evidence of an actual fungal infection.

Unfortunately "chronic candida" is not a real condition (at least not in the way that wellness culture claims) and doesn't cause all these different symptoms. In 1986, responding to the sudden popularity of "candidiasis hypersensitivity syndrome" diagnoses, the American Academy of Allergy, Asthma and Immunology researched the supposed syndrome and called it "speculative and unproven," explaining that its "basic elements..." "would apply to almost all sick patients at some time," and that there's no evidence that candida is actually the cause.[33] Since that paper was published, no new research has proven that this so-called syndrome exists, and there's no evidence from randomized controlled trials (the gold standard of scientific research) to show that cutting out sugar and/or yeast is effective in treating any genuine form of candidiasis.

The myths about sugar and candida may stem from a misapplication of the research on diabetes to people without the disease. It's true that people with poorly controlled diabetes are more susceptible to yeast infections (as well as many other types of infection)—but that's probably not because sugar "feeds" candida, as is commonly thought in diet/wellness culture. Instead, it's likely because the consistently high blood sugar caused by diabetes impairs the immune system in various ways, including by damaging cells and blood vessels, and—in the case of vaginal yeast infections—triggering a cascade of events that lead the pH of the vagina to fall, potentially making the environment more hospitable for candida to proliferate.[34] So for people with diabetes, the key to candida prevention isn't cutting out all sugar or carbs, but instead regulating your blood sugar by balancing out your carb intake with other nutrients and using other, non-diet interventions, such as taking the correct dose of oral or injectable medication.

And for those *without* diabetes, there's no reason to worry that you're somehow susceptible to candida infections just because your blood sugar naturally rises in response to eating carbohydrates. For one thing, even when people without diabetes have a blood-sugar "spike," it's generally still within the clinically "normal" range—and you'd have to have consistently, significantly high blood sugar over a sustained period of time in order to experience the immune-system impairment mentioned above. (Even people who *do* have diabetes can generally avoid those sustained highs with medication and other helpful interventions.)

What's more, a number of well-conducted studies have found that sugar consumption *doesn't* seem to play a role in candida infections. A 2006 clinical study found that consuming a large amount of sugar via an oral glucose tolerance test didn't raise vaginal glucose levels, either in women with recurrent vaginal yeast infections or in a group of age-matched controls.[35] A 1999 study found that eating an even *larger* amount of sugar for a week had no effect on candida colonization of the mouth or gastrointestinal tract among a group of "healthy" participants — and there was no association between participants' habitual carbohydrate consumption (outside the diet) and oral or fecal candida levels, either.[36] And a 2017 study found that among patients with recurrent vaginal yeast infections, blood sugar levels weren't any different between people who responded to oral antifungal medication and those who didn't.[37] So if you have periodic yeast infections, it doesn't mean you have "candida overgrowth" in the wellness-culture sense of the term, or that you need to embark on a restrictive diet to cure the condition.

Although some fungal infections are very real, wellness culture has twisted and distorted them to create a new condition — "chronic candida" — that doesn't actually exist. We see this in the proliferation of websites, social media, and alternative/ integrative providers telling people that their stuffy noses, headaches, GI problems, and all sorts of other issues are caused by candida. Today there are even stool-microbiome tests that claim to diagnose "excessive" candida in the gut, despite the fact that there are no validated reference ranges for what's considered a "normal" amount of candida in the stool. The companies selling these tests are simply making up their own numbers, and often the providers who order the tests then use the results to justify prescribing diets, supplements, and other (often very expensive) treatments. When you've been bombarded with those messages, isn't it only natural to blame any symptom you may experience on the fungi supposedly running amok in your body?

Kristin, meanwhile, is no longer convinced that candida is her issue. She's sought out help from other doctors as well as a therapist, and in the process was diagnosed with an eating disorder. "Turns out, my eating disorder and depression were at fault for many of my issues," she says. And the restrictive "candida diet" she was on only exacerbated them. "I now understand that my gut health was deteriorating under that highly restrictive diet because it was perfect only in its ability to make my actual health problems worse, and trigger new problems," she says.

She also started talking to friends who'd seen the allergist who put her on that diet, and she learned some interesting things. Her friends had all gotten pretty much the same "candida" diagnosis, and the same draconian diet and other treatments. Even after realizing that chronic candida wasn't real, Kristin reluctantly kept seeing the allergist for follow-up with the environmental allergies, but she says the doctor's response to COVID was the final straw. "At our last appointment, she very clearly was anti-vaccine," Kristin says. "And I just kind of was like, Okay, we're done. We're not doing this anymore."

### Dysfunctional Medicine

For several years Jennifer, a woman in her mid-forties who lives in the Los Angeles area (who also asked that only her first name be used), struggled with common but debilitating digestive issues including constipation, bloating, and pain. By 2015, the symptoms got bad enough that she decided to see a gastroenterologist, whom she found through her insurance. The doctor did a colonoscopy and a stomach-emptying study and found that she had gastroparesis—a condition where stomach emptying is delayed, causing a slowdown in digestion—but couldn't find anything else wrong. The doctor said she only saw gastroparesis with diabetic patients, and that since Jennifer didn't have diabetes, the doctor couldn't explain why she had the condition. (Only later did Jennifer learn that disordered eating, particularly restriction, is another major cause of gastroparesis.) The doctor diagnosed her with IBS ("which is basically 'we don't know what's wrong with your gut,'" Jennifer says), and told her to eat bland, easy-to-digest foods like white bread, white rice, and soup. To Jennifer, who already had been heavily invested in wellness culture for a few years by that point, this suggestion felt appalling. She was also frustrated that the doctor made no effort to understand or explain *why* she would have gastroparesis in the first place. "I felt completely blown off," she says.

By this point, "literally my every day was consumed with suffering, with digestive problems," Jennifer says. So she sought out another provider—this time, a nurse practitioner who specialized in functional medicine.

Proponents of functional medicine define it as a new approach that avoids many of the pitfalls of the conventional medical system. Functional medicine "seeks to identify and address the root causes of disease, and views the body as one integrated system, not a collection of independent organs divided up by medical specialties," writes Mark Hyman, one of the most famous practitioners of the paradigm.[38] "It treats the whole system, not just the symptoms . . . using a systems-oriented approach and engaging both patient and practitioner in a therapeutic partnership."

This sounds great in theory, like the antidote to a problematic healthcare system that treats different medical specialties as separate silos and gives providers very little time to devote to basic exams, let alone a "therapeutic partnership." The description suggests that functional medicine might provide what many people with chronic or unexplained illnesses (myself included) are looking for and often have trouble finding in conventional medicine. It sounds like exactly what we need.

In practice, though, functional medicine is often anything but.

Take Jennifer's experience. Right off the bat, her functional-medicine NP had her sign up for one of those at-home DNA testing services to get her genetic information, which she then uploaded to a wellness website that would supposedly diagnose her with genetic conditions. In reality, this kind of genetic "diagnosis" is not evidence based. Often people have genetic variants that would seem to make them susceptible to certain diseases, but they never actually develop those conditions. Reasons why some people with a given variant develop a disease while others don't may include characteristics of the variant, the presence of other genes that compensate for the harmful mutation, and environmental triggers for disease. Researchers are still untangling how all these factors interact and influence outcomes, and there are a lot of unknowns. Direct-to-consumer testing kits tend to gloss over that complexity, leading many geneticists to caution against using them.

Jennifer's NP also ran numerous lab tests with major labs, such as Quest and Labcorp, but would interpret the results in non-standard ways. "I kept falling into the normal range for everything," Jennifer says. "But then she would look at it and go, 'well, the lab says this is normal, but as functional medicine practitioners we use a different range.'" Although her genetic and laboratory tests for celiac disease all came back negative, Jennifer's NP said she really thought the digestive issues stemmed from a gluten intolerance and referred her to a nutritionist in her office for weekly visits. The nutritionist put her on a diet that was not only gluten-free but also highly restrictive in other ways—basically an extreme version of a well-known diet that's already quite limited. All she was allowed to eat for breakfast and lunch were shakes made with their proprietary (and pricey) shake mix.

When her condition didn't improve, Jennifer was told to cut out more foods and to purchase more and more supplements, including digestive enzymes, L-glutamine, ashwagandha, rhodiola, and a special kind of vitamin C that was supposedly better than other versions of the vitamin. At first she was happy to oblige, because the NP made her feel heard and understood.

"In the beginning I really felt like I was going to get somewhere because she was paying attention to me, and my appointments with her would last forty-five minutes," Jennifer says. "It really made me feel like, wow, someone's taking me seriously." That feeling was incredibly nourishing, as it is for many people with unexplained symptoms and poorly understood chronic conditions who've felt like they were wandering in a desert of dismissal and missed diagnoses. And the power of the provider's empathy kept her going through several months of trial and error. "Even though all the things we were trying weren't working so much, I just kept thinking, well, if anyone's going to find it, it's her because she's paying attention," Jennifer says.

Soon, though, her relationship with the NP started to change. They had gone through all the tests that were covered by her insurance, and the NP began recommending out-of-pocket tests that cost hundreds of dollars, which Jennifer didn't want to do. The diet and supplement regimen was also becoming harder and harder to manage, and Jennifer felt like she was failing. Then she had another bad flareup of her digestive issues—except this time, it was accompanied by sharp, localized abdominal pain that wouldn't go away. When she mentioned this to the NP, she says the provider responded, "Well, when your whole system is inflamed, you're going to have pain—that's just how it is." Suddenly the person who had made her feel so heard and understood was just another practitioner dismissing her pain.

That's when she decided she was done with the functional-medicine approach and sought out yet another doctor—this time, a mainstream physician who specialized in digestive disorders.

On the first visit, this new gastroenterologist palpated her belly, which none of the other providers had done. He quickly located the sore spot and thought maybe it was her gallbladder, so he sent her for an ultrasound the following morning. What they found was far worse: it turned out to be a tumor in her pancreas. From there, things happened quickly. She was referred to Cedars-Sinai in Los Angeles. She had surgery, and the doctors identified the tumor as a very rare and aggressive type called a desmoid tumor, which affects only about two to four in a million people per year.[39] She had the surgery the day before her thirty-eighth birthday, and the surgeon told her that because the tumor was located on her pancreas and interfering with critical blood vessels, he was sure that if they hadn't removed it she wouldn't have made it to forty-five.

"If I had continued with the functional-medicine crap, I would have died because my tumor never would have been found," she says.

Of course a different functional-medicine practitioner might not have missed the tumor, but Jennifer's experience highlights what seems to be a pervasive issue with functional medicine, and with wellness practitioners more broadly: many of these supposedly "holistic" providers get laser-focused on what they think is at the root of a person's problem and overlook basic aspects of patient care and diagnostics. In a patient complaining of sharp, persistent abdominal pain, palpating the abdomen ought to be a standard part of the workup. Locating the area of the pain is arguably an essential part of "treating the whole person" and "finding the root cause." Yet in too many cases, the "root cause" seems to be predetermined.

"It's almost like they're so trained in taking all those vague symptoms and attributing them to gluten or whatever that it doesn't seem to really occur to them to look outside of that box," Jennifer says of her NP and other functional-medicine providers.

Again, despite the common wellness-culture claims that Western medicine is "one size fits all" and emphasizes "popping pills," many functional- and alternative-medicine providers take a one-size-fits-all, pill-promoting approach, too—it just might look a bit different on the surface. Instead of prescribing pharmaceuticals, which at least are evaluated for safety and efficacy before going to market, they prescribe supplements, which are barely regulated. Instead of pinpointing a genuine disease as the cause of a person's symptoms, they might blame gluten (or dairy, or "leaky gut," or "adrenal fatigue") and recommend a restrictive diet. Even the diet can function in a sense like a magic pill, framed as the key to treating all manner of disparate ailments, from the common and everyday—headaches, fatigue—to rarer and more serious conditions. Functional medicine talks of unifying theories of disease, "critical imbalances that are at the root of all illness." And for people with multiple chronic conditions treated by different specialists in a siloed medical system without any coordination of care, it can be wildly appealing to think that one of these "critical imbalances" could account for all of their unexplained and confoundingly diverse symptoms. It's completely understandable why people in this situation are attracted to the promises of functional medicine and other complementary and alternative practices.

This one-size-fits-all approach might be a function of wellness-culture providers being trained in specific treatment methods and ways of conceptualizing illness. Functional-medicine doctors, naturopaths, and the like are taught to see diet as a major cause of disease and food and supplements as first-line treatments, so that's exactly what they turn to. This training effect is an issue to some extent no matter what field of healthcare—or field in general—you happen to be in: When all you have is a hammer, as the saying goes, everything looks like a nail. (And when the nail doesn't go in as expected, wellness practitioners often hammer harder, pushing even more food restrictions, supplements, and unproven practices.)

But there could be something more insidious at play, too, and that is profit motive: diagnosing virtually everyone you meet with a condition that isn't recognized by mainstream medicine, and then prescribing an elaborate food and supplement protocol to "treat" it, helps keep people coming back for appointments (which may or may not be covered by insurance) for months or years into the future. Indeed, a lovely and well-intentioned former mentor of mine, who practiced as both a dietitian and naturopathic doctor, once explained to me that putting clients on naturopathic protocols made for a much more robust private practice than simply giving them standard nutrition recommendations.

Granted, providers deserve to make a living, and it's hard to fault a micro-business owner for trying to figure out ways to stay afloat. And of course there are profit motives in conventional medicine as well—particularly in the U.S., where healthcare is considered a private rather than a public good. Yet the approaches to healing that are much vaunted in wellness culture—integrative, functional, complementary, "holistic"—are often held out as being alternatives to a profit-hungry conventional medical system, when in some ways they're no different. The real distinction is that in many cases they simply don't work as well, or at all.

### When Food Cures Fail

Asher Pandjiris is a psychotherapist who specializes in eating disorders, trauma, and navigating chronic illness, and a person who lives with two major chronic illnesses themselves. They're insightful and warm while also seeming very cool, with an artistic background and a bunch of tattoos. At age fourteen they were diagnosed with Crohn's disease, an autoimmune disorder that causes chronic inflammation of the gastrointestinal tract, which can result in symptoms including diarrhea, abdominal pain, and even malnutrition. Pandjiris received standard treatment, including medication, and got their Crohn's disease to a place where it was fairly well managed. But they still had intense abdominal symptoms flaring up on and off that conventional medical providers couldn't explain. "The Western medical world was like, 'I think you're fine,' or 'this is all in your head,' or 'look, the colonoscopy was all clear, it's good,' " they said.

This went on for years, with conventional doctors dismissing Pandjiris's lingering pain as just part of the Crohn's disease that they would have to live with for the rest of their life. They went through phases of despair and periods of thinking "fuck this, I'm just going to do whatever I want to do with my body." It wasn't until, at age twenty-seven, they had a growth literally protruding from their abdomen that a GI doctor recognized that it probably was something more than Crohn's and had them evaluated for endometriosis. When Pandjiris got that diagnosis, it was a huge relief to finally be able to identify a cause for the pelvic pain that had persisted long after their Crohn's disease was well managed. But by that point they were already feeling abandoned by the Western medical system, and they'd embarked on a path that would take them deep into the heart of wellness culture.

It started soon before they were diagnosed with endometriosis, when their symptoms were particularly acute. They decided to try acupuncture, thinking it would help with pain relief, which it did to some extent. But over the course of their sessions, the acupuncturist observed that Pandjiris's other symptoms weren't really going away and suggested that they consult with a naturopathic doctor or a nutritionist. And when they did start working with those other practitioners, Pandjiris went deeper and deeper into alternative-medicine protocols. The path can lead to an ever-growing list of supplements and tinctures, dietary restrictions and "superfoods," esoteric specialists and nonstandard blood tests that aren't supported by good scientific evidence or covered by insurance. Over the years Pandjiris lived in several major metropolitan areas around the U.S.—San Francisco, Chicago, Los Angeles, New York—and they consulted with alternative-medicine providers in all those cities. A recurring theme was the idea that they needed to get off

"Western meds" and onto a diet that would supposedly cure them completely of their chronic illnesses. "I was told, 'you can heal this straight-up with food,'" Pandjiris says.

In fact, alternative- and integrative-medicine approaches often encourage an extreme fixation on food that can easily trigger disordered eating. For one thing, restricting access to particular foods is often a surefire way to make those foods irresistible, driving many people to feel out of control around them when they inevitably do come into contact with them again. The resulting restrict-binge or restrict-rebound cycle can exacerbate the very symptoms that the diet was meant to cure, in a way that never would have happened if food hadn't been restricted in the first place. And it's not simply a matter of having more "willpower" to resist the off-limits foods; in most cases our bodies and brains are actually programmed to override those restrictions and get their needs met, as I discuss in *Anti-Diet*. For the rare people who can stick with a restrictive diet for any length of time, the risk of spiraling into anorexia or orthorexia is high.

Pandjiris was one of the latter group who did stick with the restrictive diet—and they still found that it wasn't helpful. Looking back, they now see that a lot of the things on the diet— such as juicing, raw foods, large quantities of fish oil—were incredibly hard on their gut, which is not ideal when you're struggling with digestive problems and pelvic pain. And then there were all the supplements. "I was being prescribed heavy-duty amounts of really intense probiotics, and so many supplements that in retrospect I understand were making it hard for me to digest the food and were really wreaking havoc on my body," they say. Very few of their practitioners, if any, suggested easily digestible foods like white bread or white rice, which they now know are gentler on their system. Although they were never told by a practitioner to try a celery-juice cleanse, they found that it always popped up in searches for Crohn's disease, often leading back to the Medical Medium. But it wasn't just online;

numerous friends and other well-meaning people in Pandjiris's life recommended celery juice. "They said, 'look, I really think this could help you'—and by help me they meant cure me," Pandjiris says, though there is no cure for their conditions.

The heart of the diet, though, was eliminating foods. The types of foods to cut out depended on which condition was being targeted at the time, but they remember that if the endometriosis was in the crosshairs, they were told in no uncertain terms, "you MUST have a plant-based diet, you MUST not eat eggs, you MUST not eat gluten." They were put on low-FODMAP diets—diets low in the types of carbohydrates that may trigger intestinal pain for some people, namely fermentable oligosaccharides, disaccharides, monosaccharides and polyols—and "autoimmune protocol" diets.

Pandjiris would dutifully follow these diets to the letter, but nothing seemed to work. And when they went back to these practitioners after several months to say that they felt pretty much the same—if not worse, because they were so stressed out about food—the providers didn't seem to know what to do. "People would often just be confused and confounded by me, as if I was some sort of anomaly," they say. It seemed like the practitioners were implying that all their other patients were cured by these interventions, and perhaps they did have many "success stories"—but it's also hard to believe they'd never seen these protocols fail. Indeed, there's no evidence from randomized controlled trials to support the use of the autoimmune protocol diet for any condition, and the low-FODMAP diet shouldn't be used long-term, even if it may potentially be helpful for short-term use in a subset of patients with inflammatory bowel diseases.[40] But the providers seemed to believe wholeheartedly in these diets, and they would grill Pandjiris: "Are you sure you're not having alcohol? Are you sure you're not having caffeine? Are you sure you're not slipping and having cheese every once in a while?" When Pandjiris assured them that they were following the diet 100 percent ("I can really do something by the book if you want me to, and I will, probably to a fault," they say), the providers seemed to be at a loss.

These providers made Pandjiris feel that they were personally responsible for healing themselves through diet and stress management, without recognizing the importance of mental health or other factors beyond their individual control. And for Pandjiris, other factors were indeed likely at play. "[There wasn't] a lot of thought about maybe what was happening with my nervous system as a result of having these conditions, in addition to having a pretty significant history of childhood trauma," they said. As discussed in Chapter 3, those kinds of life experiences can have a major impact on health outcomes, and adherence to standard wellness-culture protocols like diets and supplements generally does not alleviate stress and other, more profound aftereffects of trauma—and certainly is not a cure.

Another reason why alternative medicine was so appealing to Pandjiris was that it felt more welcoming of certain aspects of their identity. "Being queer and non-binary and being in a community with other queer, non-binary trans people, the healthcare system is, for the most part, really pathologizing of our bodies," Pandjiris says. "And I think that in lots of marginalized communities, these alternative spaces do initially feel more welcoming, more empowering." Though Pandjiris acknowledges that they have a tremendous amount of privilege as a white, relatively thin person, they've often felt that alternative health was more in alignment with their values and more hospitable to them as someone with a body that Western medicine tends to treat as weird or abnormal. That alternative providers ended up failing Pandjiris in many ways is especially disheartening given the promise of acceptance and compassion those providers had seemed to hold out.

Indeed, the fact that alternative-medicine spaces offering ineffective and often harmful "cures" are the most welcoming to marginalized people—and are frequently the only places many people with chronic illnesses feel we can go to have our symptoms taken seriously—is a tragedy. It's a sign of the healthcare system's brokenness that there aren't solid, evidence-based treatments to offer people in these situations, and that instead those of us with complex and poorly understood health problems are left to wander alone in the often dangerous territory of wellness culture. Sometimes we're so desperate for healing that we try questionable therapies even when our alarm bells are going off. "Decisions like this are often portrayed as products of the patient's credulousness, her naïveté," Meghan O'Rourke writes.[41] "But the reality is that many of us are people who, faced with no good choice, shrug our way into the hands of those we don't trust in search of help."

It's important to have compassion for ourselves and others who've been drawn in by wellness culture's false promises of cures for real diseases—or by its dubious diagnoses. It's completely understandable that when you have a long history of being dismissed by doctors or failed by the healthcare system, you'd be vulnerable to falling into the wellness trap. Unfortunately, many well-meaning alternative-medicine providers end up making preexisting health problems worse by prescribing supplements and promoting and recommending unproven diets that drive some people into (or further into) disordered eating and sometimes mask far more serious problems. Most of these providers almost certainly aren't trying to do harm, it just ends up that way. But there are also many unscrupulous actors in wellness culture who deliberately prey on people's desperation. It's those scammers and snake-oil salespeople that we'll turn to next.

# CHAPTER 7

# Scams, Schemes, and Snake Oil

For a few brief, intense years, Belle Gibson was a poster girl for wellness culture. The thin, blond young mom's meteoric rise began in 2013, when she made her debut post on Instagram. From an account called @healing_belle, she shared that she had terminal brain cancer (she would later claim, without evidence, that she'd gotten the cancer from a vaccine) and was now successfully treating it through "natural" means—cutting out gluten and refined sugar, taking herbal supplements, using unproven and dangerous methods like oxygen therapy and colonics, and engaging in many other controversial practices. She said that while she'd been given only months to live, she was thriving four years later thanks solely to these alternative treatments.

The story hit a nerve with a wellness-hungry user base, and Gibson's audience soon swelled to tens of thousands of followers. People flocked to her page, many of them suffering from cancer and chronic illnesses, seeking advice and guidance—and she seemed happy to deliver. As she wrote in one post, "I gave up on conventional treatment when it was making my cancer more aggressive and started treating myself naturally. I have countless times helped others do the same, along with leading them down natural therapy for everything from fertility, depression, bone damage and other types of cancer."[1]

In July of 2014, she announced on Instagram that her brain

cancer had returned and spread to her blood, spleen, uterus, and liver. Although in different circumstances that might have been a red flag to her audience that her unconventional treatment methods weren't working, in Gibson's case that argument didn't seem to register. By that point, she and her brand, The Whole Pantry, had become enormously popular in her native Australia and around the world. She'd launched an iPhone app by the same name in August of 2013, and just a few months later it was voted Apple's Best Food and Drink App of the year, and the second most popular iPhone app in the world. She'd landed a major book deal with Penguin Australia.

In the months following her announcement of the metastasis, Apple revealed that The Whole Pantry would be one of only a few apps featured on its new watch, and Penguin Australia released her cookbook—a gorgeous, 250-page tome filled not just with supposedly health-enhancing recipes but also with advice on beauty, gut health, weight loss, and even how to make your own cleaning products. Gibson's story of healing from cancer was prominently featured in the introduction (despite the fact that she was apparently now suffering a relapse).

Granted, some in the media looked askance at Gibson's claims. "I always thought the fact that she recovered from terminal brain cancer via natural remedies to be bullshit," says Kate Spies, now a wellness-media executive in the U.S. Spies, who is from Australia and was working as a journalist at the popular women's lifestyle site *Mamamia* at the height of Gibson's fame, said, "I just did not believe that for a second, and I think large parts of the population in the media didn't." But those skeptics notwithstanding, Gibson still got glowing coverage in major media outlets, which praised her app, her looks, her bravery in ostensibly eschewing conventional medicine to find healing. She received a "Fun, Fearless Female" social media award from Australian *Cosmopolitan*. Her book became a sensation in Australia, and she jetted around on national and international speaking engagements to promote it. It was set to be published in the UK by a Penguin imprint there, and in the U.S. by an imprint of Simon & Schuster. As journalists Beau Donelly and Nick Toscano wrote in 2017, "Emerging from obscurity, Gibson had gained traction in Australia, America, and the UK in just 18 months, becoming one of the most famous wellness personalities in the world."[2]

Like many wellness influencers, Gibson didn't have advanced degrees or professional expertise in the subjects she wrote about. She had no post-secondary education in nutrition or recipe development, let alone cancer treatment. She'd dropped out of high school at age sixteen. Shortly after that, she'd gotten a job in a call center at a private health insurance company, where she listened to details of clients' medical problems day in and day out — despite still being a minor and lacking health-related credentials. To her credit, she didn't publicly claim to have any qualifications other than her own lived experience; according to her Instagram bio, she was a "gamechanger with brain cancer + a food obsession."[3] Her audience didn't seem to mind that her work with The Whole Pantry was based solely on her personal story.

Unfortunately, that story turned out to be completely false. In reality, Belle Gibson was one of the biggest wellness scammers in recent history.

It all started to unravel because she'd been claiming to give large sums of money to charity, variously alleging that she donated "all profits" from app sales and 25 percent either of her company's profits, or of app profits to organizations devoted to health, the environment, and education; elsewhere she is reported to have said that "100 per cent of app sales for one week would be donated to the parents of a boy with terminal brain cancer."[4] When that money never materialized, people began asking questions. In 2015, as reporters for the Australian newspaper *The Age*, Donelly and Toscano started digging into her purported contributions and found that Gibson had solicited donations from her 200,000 followers "in the name of at least five charities that have no record of receiving money from her."[5] In response, The Whole Pantry posted a statement on social media claiming that the company was having cash-flow problems, and that it would make the promised contributions once its books were in order. The backlash on social media was swift, and followers became increasingly agitated as they saw their critical comments disappear, deleted by Gibson or her team.

Soon after *The Age*'s reporting about Gibson's false claims of charitable donations, people close to her started coming forward to say they had their doubts about other aspects of her story. Looking to do damage control, Gibson went to a journalist and confessed: not only had she failed to donate the money she promised to charity, but she also *never even really had cancer.* She'd made up the whole thing.

"None of it's true," she admitted to *Australian Women's Weekly*, in an article from the May 2015 issue headlined "My Lifelong Struggle with the Truth."[6] The doctor who she claimed diagnosed her with cancer, Mark Johns of the Peter MacCallum Cancer Centre in Melbourne, doesn't appear ever to have existed; there are no records of anyone by that name having been employed by the cancer center or even being registered to practice medicine in Australia. Gibson had lied about her age, too: she actually is three years younger than she'd claimed to be, meaning that at the time of her supposed brain cancer diagnosis in 2009 she was only seventeen, and when her worldwide wellness empire finally crumbled she was all of twenty-three.

People who'd been duped by her were understandably furious, and they often took to the Internet to speak out. Gibson was publicly excoriated in the media and on social media in a way that's all too familiar to anyone who's been online in the past ten years, but her public shaming was perhaps even more intense than is typical because of the sheer brazenness of her deceit. She received an avalanche of death threats. Others out for vengeance fell just short of that, threatening to physically harm her. Her home address was published online (a form of Internet attack known as doxing), which gave the threats legitimacy. The name of her young son's school was revealed, putting him in danger. By the time her case went before a federal judge, in 2017,[7] she'd already been tried and convicted in the court of public opinion.

Gibson's story is extreme, to be sure. Few people lie as flagrantly as she did, and even fewer reach her level of success based entirely on lies. This saga is captivating perhaps because it's rare.

Still, many elements of it are all too common in wellness culture, even if the lies are typically less extravagant: The lionization of a young, beautiful person with no credentials; the outlandish claims about the healing powers of food and "natural" remedies; the virality of her message and the way she quickly spun it off into lucrative business deals; the role of social media in both her rise and her downfall; and the failure of conventional media to fact-check her claims. Although her scam took place almost a decade ago, in many ways it's still perfectly relevant to contemporary wellness culture—perhaps even more so today, given that scams are having a moment in the current climate of mis- and disinformation.

Yet Gibson and all the other wellness scammers plying their trade today are in many ways working from a playbook developed in a bygone era. To understand the landscape of wellness-culture scams today, it helps to go back to its roots in the age when "snake oil" was meant literally.

### Snake Oil and Medicine Shows

In the late 1800s, an American entrepreneur named Clark Stanley became known as the Rattlesnake King. Stanley, a former cowboy, claimed to have studied with Hopi medicine men and learned "the secret of making the Snake Oil Medicine" that the tribe supposedly used for all manner of aches and pains.[8] He said he improved upon their formula in order to create his product, Clark Stanley's Snake Oil Liniment, which he marketed for numerous conditions including nerve pain (neuralgia), rheumatoid arthritis (rheumatism), toothache, sore throat, and "bites of animals, insects, and reptiles."

In fact, his story and claims about his product were all completely fabricated.

The nineteenth century was the era of medicine shows, where various unskilled healers and hucksters traveled the country hawking patent medicines—those "cure-all" nostrums we discussed in Chapter 2, which in reality had little to no effect on the conditions they were purported to treat. Nineteenth-century medicine shows used entertainment as marketing to sell patent medicines to the public. So-called pitchmen—because they were indeed almost universally men—traveled with groups of circus folks, vaudeville actors, and even minstrel-show performers, whose racist acts became popular among mostly white audiences. Often these groups would perform shows unrelated to the medicine, and then the sales pitch would come at the end, once the audience was warmed up by the entertainment. Some pitches involved an audience plant pretending to be physically disabled in some way, and then after the patent medicine was administered they would suddenly, "miraculously," be able to walk or see, which generally provoked a huge response and a deluge of sales.

Stereotypes about disability and race were prevalent in many medicine shows, but one kind in particular was built pretty much entirely around racist tropes: shows that sold "herbal" remedies advertised as having been created by Native Americans. The best-known were those mounted by the Kickapoo Indian Medicine Company, the brainchild of a couple of white guys named John

Healy and Charles Bigelow, who'd been working in the patent-medicine trade for years and were searching for the next big thing.[9] In 1881 they started manufacturing remedies that they claimed were given to them by Kickapoo medicine men—a story chosen because Healy found the tribe's name amusing. Nineteenth-century patent-medicine promoters had been capitalizing for years on a stereotype of Native Americans as natural healers, "Mother Nature's physicians." Healy and Bigelow marketed their products as "secret" concoctions of herbs, when in fact they were purchased from drug wholesalers. The whole operation was steeped in fake Native American lore, and in the beginning Healy and Bigelow included a few Indigenous people as background actors in their shows. As their operation grew, they began hiring Native performers by the dozen to stage scenes, speeches, and faux ceremonies, which were interspersed with other acts: vaudeville, brass bands, and carnival performances. By the late 1880s, Kickapoo had the largest and most prosperous medicine show of the era, with as many as one hundred different traveling companies that crisscrossed the country.[10]

Healy and Bigelow's success inspired numerous competitors who claimed some connection to Native American culture (most of whom had none to speak of, with the exception of a few Native proprietors). Native American–themed medicine shows were all the rage, and people across the patent-medicine industry wanted in on the act. This may have been the inspiration for Stanley, the Rattlesnake King, to claim that his snake oil was a recipe from Hopi medicine men—even though the idea of snake oil itself most likely came via other channels.

Between 1849 and 1882, thousands of Chinese immigrants came to the United States to work in the booming railroad industry (and unsurprisingly were paid low wages relative to their white counterparts).[11] With them, these workers brought a traditional pain remedy from home: snake oil. Made from Chinese water snakes, whose fat is naturally high in omega-3 fatty acids from feeding on fish, this original snake oil was actually somewhat effective at treating pain and inflammatory joint conditions like arthritis and bursitis. Chinese railroad workers would rub the oil on their joints after a hard day's work, and some reportedly shared it with the Americans who worked alongside them. Soon word started to spread about snake oil, which may have been how Stanley first heard about it. But anti-Chinese racism and xenophobia were strong at the time, and it's likely that snake oil's origins would have been seen as less romantic—and less marketable—than a made-up claim about a remedy procured from Native Americans.

Stanley's claims didn't have to be truthful to be believed. His medicine show was sensational: at the 1893 World's Columbian Exposition in Chicago, he pulled a live rattlesnake out of a bag, sliced it open, and dunked it in a vat of boiling water, no doubt to the shock and amazement of the audience. He then skimmed the fat off the top of the vat and poured it into bottles right in front of the people who lined up to receive it. What they (and probably even Stanley) didn't know is that rattlesnake oil is largely devoid of omega-3 fats and is pretty much useless for pain, let alone for the other conditions Stanley claimed it could cure, such as sprains, bruises, and frostbite. This also wasn't the snake oil normally sold in Stanley's bottles—the attendees at his live show got a special batch that the mountebank likely never replicated outside that setting.

In fact, the pre-bottled "snake oil" that Stanley sold in huge quantities contained no actual oil from snakes at all, rattlers or otherwise. As testing in 1916 showed, it was a mix of mineral oil, beef fat, capsicum, and "possibly a trace of camphor and turpentine."[12] Stanley also never publicly mentioned Chinese snake oil, choosing instead to stick to a more marketable but almost certainly false story about the product's origins.

Faux snake oil like the kind Stanley sold was almost certainly ineffective, but at the time, "conventional" medicine wasn't much better. In fact, it wasn't even truly conventional yet. "In the nineteenth century, before you really have a professionalized medical establishment, there is a more permeable boundary between so-called legitimate medical practitioners and those who are practicing a kind of alternative medicine because the mainstream is not yet formed," says Natalia Mehlman Petrzela, the historian of fitness and wellness culture. "Our boundaries of what's legitimate and what is alternative have shifted over time." Germ theory was in its infancy, and even trained doctors only had ineffective tools in their toolbox.

It's no wonder patent medicine was attractive to consumers, its appeal enhanced by purveyors' exploitation, in their marketing, of the limitations of the medical system. Today's wellness industry often likewise positions itself in opposition to conventional medicine. Patent-medicine makers pointed out that treatment by doctors often produced intense side effects, while their remedies were supposedly gentle—and far cheaper than medical care. And when doctors cautioned seriously ill patients against using patent medicines because they might delay proper treatment and worsen outcomes, manufacturers lashed back, saying that doctors were just trying to limit competition and keep all the business for themselves—the same rhetoric that shows up in many wellness scams and medical conspiracy theories today.

### Vulnerability to Scams

It's probably no accident that Belle Gibson's epic wellness con centered around cancer, or that some of the most outrageous claims about wellness products have to do with preventing or curing cancer. In many ways people are especially vulnerable to mis- and disinformation about cancer because for all the incredible advances medicine has made in treatment, it's not guaranteed to work and the side effects are often brutal. There are also many misconceptions about the disease. More than a third of Americans—a staggering 35 percent—erroneously believe that cancer can be cured using alternative therapies alone, according to a nationally representative survey of 4,012 U.S. adults in 2020 by the American Society of Clinical Oncology (ASCO).[13] (For the record, numerous studies have found that people who use alternative cancer therapies instead of conventional treatment actually have an increased risk of death, even when the severity of their cancer is taken into account.*) That false belief is likely driven in part by the fact that most people don't know

---

* A study with five-year survival rate as one metric found that on average, using alternative treatments alone was associated with more than double the risk of death. The risk was far greater in cases of colorectal cancer—people who used only alternative medicine were more than 4.5 times more likely to die—and greater still for breast cancer: patients were nearly six times more likely to die. (Skyler B. Johnson et al., "Use of Alternative Medicine for Cancer and Its Impact on Survival," *JNCI: Journal of the National Cancer Institute* 110, no. 1 [January 1, 2018]: 121–24, https://doi.org/10.1093/jnci/djx145.) Another study found that among patients with curable cancers, those who used complementary medicine—herbs and botanicals, vitamins and minerals, traditional Chinese medicine, homeopathy, naturopathy, and specialized diets, in *addition* to at least one conventional treatment—were significantly more likely to refuse other recommended conventional cancer treatments. These patients had about twice the risk of death as those who used conventional treatments alone. This is especially concerning given that previous studies have found that between 48 and 88 percent of people with cancer report using complementary and alternative medicine as part of their therapy. (Skyler B. Johnson et al., "Complementary Medicine, Refusal of Conventional Cancer Therapy, and Survival among Patients with Curable Cancers," *JAMA Oncology* 4, no. 10 [October 1, 2018]: 1375, https://doi.org/10.1001/jamaoncol.2018.2487.)

where to go for reliable information about cancer: 63 percent of ASCO survey respondents agreed with the statements "I'm not sure which sources to trust when it comes to information about what causes cancer" and "it is hard to know the most important things to do to reduce my risk of getting cancer."

But this problem goes far beyond cancer. Today we struggle to trust all kinds of information about health and wellness — not to mention information about science, politics, and the world more generally. Misinformation abounds online, spreading faurther and faster than the truth. And shared truth has largely broken down, abetted by social media algorithms, filter bubbles, and attacks from right-wing media. The postmodernism that has been influential in many corners of academia (and that formed the core of my studies in Rhetoric as an undergraduate back in the early 2000s) may also have played a role. Though some postmodernist thinkers have made important observations about how social factors (such as the forces keeping women out of the medical field) affect scientific research and understanding, postmodern critiques of science can also be taken to extremes (for example, positing that science has no more claim to certainty than alternative paradigms like astrology and witchcraft) or weaponized (arguing that climate scientists are irredeemably biased and that the evidence on climate change is therefore suspect).[14] In this "post-truth" context, emotions and beliefs often hold more sway than facts, and the concept of "the truth" is replaced with the much squishier notion of "your truth."

Contributing to this shift is the breakdown of confidence in institutions. As I write this, Americans' average level of trust in fourteen major institutions is at an all-time low, according to a 2022 Gallup poll.[15] The survey found that only 38 percent of people said they have either a great deal or quite a lot of confidence in the medical system, down six percentage points from the previous year. This lack of trust is in many ways understandable: The CDC, for example, made numerous missteps in its handling of COVID-19, including bungling the rollout of testing kits, bowing to political pressure from the Trump White House to change or withhold certain public health guidance, and underestimating the threat posed by variants. In the wake of a 2022 internal investigation into the agency's COVID-19 failures, CDC director Rochelle Walensky said in a video to employees that "we are responsible for some pretty dramatic, pretty public mistakes from testing to data to communications" and called for the CDC to be reorganized to better address public health.[16] Less recently, the FDA made a grave regulatory error in its decision to approve the opioid OxyContin for chronic pain, helping to ignite the opioid crisis. The agency had previously approved the drug for short-term use based on strong evidence for that indication, but in 2001 it gave in to pressure from drugmaker Purdue Pharma to revise the drug's label to say that OxyContin was now approved for patients with moderate to severe pain requiring "a continuous around-the-clock analgesic for an extended period of time," despite no new science to support the safety or efficacy of long-term use.[17] The revised label included the most stringent safety warning that the FDA could give for an approved drug, and the agency also worked with Purdue to come up with a plan for preventing abuse of the medication. Nevertheless, the revised labeling ultimately cleared the way for OxyContin's increased use, and as *60 Minutes* reported in 2019, "an internal document shows the company was jubilant about the labeling change."[18] Federal agencies later responded to the opioid crisis by issuing stringent 2016 prescription guidelines, which some doctors and patients say has led to "a culture of austerity around opioids" and "a crisis of untreated pain."[19]

When institutions tasked with looking out for public health are on shaky ground, it's no wonder that many people lose faith in them or cease to trust them altogether.

Institutional failures (coupled with the neoliberal belief in personal responsibility previously discussed) can give the impression that we're solely responsible for our own safety—that no one is looking out for us, and that we need to "do our own research" instead of trusting experts and entities that we suspect are only out for profit and not invested in our well-being. Indeed, one can feel compelled to try to become an "expert in everything," as writer and sociologist Tressie McMillan Cottom puts it.[20] In the realm of wellness, this happens when those who are not healthcare professionals feel the need to try to analyze scientific data and anecdotal evidence in order to make their own decisions about vaccines, masking, kids' school attendance, treatments for chronic illnesses. It happens elsewhere in contemporary life as well, compounded by a social media environment that prods us to publish our "take" on every social issue, pushing everyday people to release statements and policy prescriptions as if we were politicians.

Ironically, though, attempting to be an expert in everything makes us even more vulnerable to scams, because scammers tend to prey on people's overconfidence in their own abilities. "A citizen consumer who thinks he or she is an expert in all manner of everyday decisions is the perfect mark for an endless string of scams," McMillan Cottom writes. For example, a 2022 study among a nationally representative sample in China found that people who were overconfident about their financial knowledge were more likely to believe fraudulent claims about an investment opportunity.[21] Getting scammed doesn't necessarily mean being the victim of illegal activity, however; scams can be legal but still exploitative, deceptive, or misleading, like snake oil and other wellness products that make false promises and fail to deliver. Because there's no meaningful oversight of health claims made online or on dietary-supplement bottles, purveyors of wellness-culture products and programs—from herbal tinctures and essential oils to weight-loss plans and supposed cures for chronic disease—can make wild assertions with no evidence to back them up, deceiving the public in order to enrich themselves.

Given that we're living in an environment that's ripe for scams and that we actually *aren't* able to be experts in everything, how can we sort through all the information that's constantly flowing through our feeds to figure out what's trustworthy?

A good place to start is a method that's taught in many media-literacy courses called SIFT, developed by University of Washington research scientist Mike Caulfield, who studies how digital information literacy can help combat mis- and disinformation. SIFT stands for its four steps:

Stop.
Investigate the source.
Find better coverage.
Trace claims, quotes, and media to the original context.[22]

SIFT is meant to help people think twice before reflexively sharing or acting upon unverified information. The process involves quickly moving away from the actual content of the misinformation and focusing on the context, so that you're not wasting precious time trying to dissect dubious sources—because that's exactly what peddlers of disinformation want you to do. "The goal of disinformation is to capture attention, and critical thinking is deep attention," Caulfield wrote in 2018. "Whenever you give your attention to a bad actor, you allow them to steal your attention from better treatments of an issue, and give them the opportunity to warp your perspective."[23] So instead of doing a deep dive into misinformation to try to understand it from the inside—which is what we might traditionally view as critical thinking—you're better off seeking out other, more credible sources to put the information into context.

In 2021, Caulfield walked a *New York Times* writer through the SIFT process using an Instagram post from anti-vaccine activist (and number two on the Disinformation Dozen list) Robert F. Kennedy Jr.[24] After reading Kennedy's post—which falsely linked a certain vaccine to cancer—Caulfield quickly left Instagram and headed over to Google to look up his name. Within 15 seconds, he had found a reputable source identifying Kennedy as an anti-vax activist who promotes the scientifically discredited claim that vaccines cause autism. "Is Robert F. Kennedy Jr. the best, unbiased source on information about a vaccine? I'd argue no," Caulfield told the *Times* writer. "And that's good enough to know we should probably just move on."

In that example, Caulfield only had to get to the "I" in SIFT—investigate the source—to know he was ready to dismiss Kennedy's Instagram post. In similar situations, as with Belle Gibson's cancer claims or Clark Stanley's bombastic assertions about snake oil's ability to cure all ills, investigating the source might have been enough to deter many people as well: Gibson was a young woman without any healthcare credentials making implausible claims based purely on her own experience, and Stanley was a literal snake-oil salesman, in the era when that term developed the negative connotations it has today.

In other cases, you might have to go through the full SIFT process to spot a scam. To find better coverage (the "F" in SIFT), you'd want to look beyond social media and the person's website—getting outside the echo chamber where everyone is reflexively supporting their claims—to see if any reputable sources say the same thing. Of course "reputable" can feel like a tricky concept these days, but as mentioned previously, mainstream news outlets are held to journalistic standards and also can be sued for making false or unsubstantiated reports, so they're often a good source for cross-referencing claims that seem too good to be true. They also tend to be very interested in health and wellness trends and would likely be all over it if there really was, say, an effective alternative to chemotherapy for cancer—so if they're *not* covering something, it can be a sign that the product or practice doesn't pass muster. Major organizations devoted to particular diseases, such as the American Cancer Society or the American Heart Association, also can be good sources for checking alternative-health claims, though their guidance around food and weight is often rooted in diet culture. And although many high school teachers won't let students cite it as a source, Wikipedia is a surprisingly good jumping-off point for a critical analysis of wellness claims, as it includes links to relevant scientific references and skeptical commentary about common practices in alternative and integrative medicine.

Finally, the last step in SIFT is to trace claims, quotes, and media to their original context. To do this for potential wellness scams, you'd look at whether there are any scientific studies or other sources cited, and whether those references actually seem to support the claims—or whether citations are being taken out of context (or entirely fabricated, as is occasionally the case). And if there *aren't* any legitimate outside sources cited, that can be a red flag, too—such as when the Medical Medium says he has it on authority from "the Spirit" that drinking celery juice every day can cure all manner of chronic diseases, but that science hasn't yet caught up with this knowledge. When a source makes a sensational claim but offers no way to fact-check it, that may be a sign of manipulation.

With the SIFT method in mind, let's look at another category of scams that have proliferated in wellness spaces in the past few decades.

## Multilevel Marketing

In June of 1983, Gary Young was convicted for the first time of practicing medicine without a license. At the time he ran an herb shop and nutrition center in Spokane, Washington, with his then wife. In 1982, the couple had lost a newborn daughter, in a tragic turn of events: Young, a proponent of alternative medicine, believed that underwater birth could prevent disease, and he delivered the baby in a whirlpool bath at a health club he operated, leaving her submerged for almost an hour. The county coroner later said that the newborn probably would have lived had she been delivered conventionally.[25] No charges were brought, but the circumstances were suspicious enough that authorities decided to start looking into Young. Two undercover officers contacted him, posing as a couple looking for alternative methods of delivery of a child they said they were expecting. Young gave them prenatal counseling and offered to be present at the birth, as well as to monitor the "pregnant" officer's blood and make nutritional prescriptions. He also made recommendations for treating a family member's cancer through alternative medicine rather than surgery and chemotherapy. He proposed testing the blood of the officer posing as the expectant father "to determine body deterioration, organ malfunction, and compatibility for food and food supplements," according to court records obtained by *Business Insider*.[26]

Young had no medical training, and no valid credentials in the health and wellness field — he had attended three unaccredited schools, including one run by a shady character who had himself been convicted of practicing medicine without a license and several other crimes. When Young produced a blood-testing syringe, which the male officer brought to the bathroom to draw his own blood to be tested (Young having explained that he did not himself take blood samples), he was arrested.

As a thirty-three-year-old white man, Young's encounter with the police was a lot less tragic than it otherwise might have been. He didn't have to do jail time, and he was sentenced only to probation. That, and he had to promise not to practice medicine in Washington or any other U.S. state again. Though there are many issues with the American criminal-justice system, it's probably an overall benefit to society that someone like Young — who'd already had a person die on his watch — would be stopped from practicing medicine.

Except he didn't stop.

Prior to sentencing, Young moved to a small town in San Diego County, California, on the Mexican border. There, he told probation officers, he started working as a "nutritional consultant" employed by an MD who split his time between California and Mexico. In July 1983, Young asked for permission to travel with this doctor between the two countries and was told to stay put until the California probation department could review his request.[27] In a September 1983 report, a California probation officer expressed concerns "regarding the possibility that the defendant is continuing his 'medical practices' in Mexico and, therefore, might be subjecting Mexican citizens to potential harm." The officer suspected that Young was looking to flee the country in order to try to "elude detection and prosecution" for continuing to practice medicine without a license.

It appears that that's exactly what he was doing. While he did set up a health shop on the U.S. side of the border, his real work seemed to be in Mexico, where he opened a clinic called the Younger Life and Health Education and Research Foundation (*Clinica Vida y Salud*, later rebranded as the Rosarita Beach Clinic). The clinic claimed to treat degenerative diseases—primarily cancer, for which it claimed to have an 85 percent success rate, as well as multiple sclerosis, diabetes, and cardiovascular disease—via a cornucopia of alternative therapies, such as detox diets, colonics, and supplements. The clinic also used dubious diagnostic methods, including a "blood crystallization" test that apparently couldn't distinguish between human blood and that of other species, as a reporter for the *Los Angeles Times* found in 1987 when he submitted samples for analysis that were actually taken from a cat and a chicken.[28] In a line that could have been lifted out of Belle Gibson's book three decades later, a clinic brochure promised that clients "will learn how to rid the body of tissue-destroying toxins and how to rejuvenate the organs, glands, and tissues to repair and rebuild." The brochure listed Young as the clinic's medical director, and said that he had moved to Mexico to escape "harassment from the orthodox medical profession."

Apparently that wasn't the only organization he was trying to escape: he also skipped out on his probation meetings and disconnected his phone. His probation record from November 1983 listed his status as "absconder" and recommended issuing a bench warrant for his arrest.

That arrest came nearly five years later, in Seattle, and this time he spent about a month in jail (after which he got another year of probation). The same year, 1988, the state of California filed a complaint against him for "unfair, deceptive, untrue and misleading advertising and unlawful, unfair and fraudulent business practices," because not only was he still claiming to be able to cure cancer and other diseases, but now he was also illegally manufacturing medical devices and selling pharmaceuticals. One of the inspectors who investigated Young's facility found that some of the drugs were dangerous enough to warrant confiscation, including sixty-one bottles of "Parasitic Bowel Cleanser Extract" and two bottles of "Thyroid 130."

The California case was ultimately settled, but Young, like a traveling snake-oil salesman, moved states again, in early 1989 — this time to Nevada. His company continued selling blends of herbs and vitamins with names like "Colon Aid" and "Liver Tone," for "detoxifying" and "cleansing." Then, just a few years later, he relocated to Utah, where he started selling oils of his own.

Today you might know Young's name from the popular multilevel-marketing company (MLM) he founded: Young Living. At first the company sold a variety of alternative-medicine products, but in the early 1990s, after the Utah move, Young Living transitioned to selling primarily essential oils. Perhaps this pivot had something to do with the fact that Young was becoming ever more distrustful of conventional medicine, and more and more drawn to increasingly obscure alternatives like oils distilled from various aromatic plants, which at the time were largely used as fragrance and flavoring agents. He'd become fascinated by the supposed medicinal properties of the oils after meeting a French lavender distiller at a holistic-health expo in California, and he'd subsequently gone to France to study distillation methods.

At the same time, as he switched to selling oils, Young also took the MLM aspect of his business to the next level. The distinguishing feature of MLMs is a business structure made up of independent distributors who sell the company's products directly to people in their own networks—friends and family, and, increasingly, social media acquaintances—and recruit other distributors under them, creating what's known as a downline. In most MLMs, directly selling the products might yield a little bit of income (if any), but the real money is in having a big downline: each new recruit typically either has to buy a bunch of products up front or pay a hefty joining fee (or both), and the person who recruited them (their "upline") gets a cut. If you draw a diagram of all the uplines and downlines, it resembles a triangle or pyramid, and indeed many critics of MLMs allege that they're pyramid schemes—scams in which each participant pays to join and then enlists several other people, earning commissions on payments made by their recruits (and the recruits of those recruits, on down the line).

A popular trope in MLMs is to say that you only need to recruit five people, and then they each recruit five people, who each recruit five more people, and so on—and then you sit back and watch the commissions roll in from your downline. In fact, it's mathematically impossible for that scheme to work for long: After only thirteen cycles, you've exceeded the entire population of the earth.[29] Pyramid schemes are illegal in most countries, not only because of that mathematical impossibility but because the last people who join—the vast majority of people, who make up the base of the pyramid—aren't able to recruit anyone, and so they lose their investment while those at the top of the pyramid profit handsomely. A 2011 report to the Federal Trade Commission (FTC) found that 99 percent of MLM participants lose money.[30] Technically, the difference between an MLM and a pyramid scheme is that MLMs have legitimate products that people can make money by selling. In practice, many former MLM distributors and critics say that MLM products are just a cover for a scam in which recruitment is the actual goal, and that only the people at the top of large downlines see any real profits. So far, however, even some of the most egregious MLMs generally aren't considered pyramid schemes in the U.S.*

------

* For example, in 2014, the FTC launched an investigation into the diet-shake and supplement company Herbalife, after a hedge-fund manager publicly accused the company of being a pyramid scheme. It found that Herbalife "deceived consumers into believing they could earn substantial money selling diet, nutritional supplement, and personal care products," required the company to pay $200 million to the victims who'd lost money, and forced them to restructure their business—but stopped short of calling them a pyramid scheme. Technically, the FTC said, "the multi-level marketing company's compensation structure was unfair because it rewards distributors for recruiting others to join and purchase products in order to advance in the marketing program, rather than in response to actual retail demand for the product, causing substantial economic injury to many of its distributors"—language that would seem to suggest that the ultimate settlement between the two parties included an agreement not to use the words "pyramid scheme." (Lesley Fair, "It's No Longer Business as Usual at Herbalife: An Inside Look at the $200 Million FTC Settlement," Federal Trade Commission blog, July 15, 2016, https://www.ftc.gov/business-guidance/blog/2016/07/its-no-longer-business-usual-herbalife-inside-look-200-million-ftc-settlement; see also Case 2:16-cv-05217, Document 1, Filed July 15, 2016, https://www.ftc.gov/system/files/documents/cases/160715herbalifecmpt.pdf). So legally, as of this writing, Herbalife is not a pyramid scheme.

Whatever you call them, one thing is clear: the entity at the very top—the company itself—profits the most from the arrangement. MLMs are a massive global industry, with $179.3 billion in retail sales in 2020.[31]

Wellness is by far the biggest category in the MLM industry, representing 36 percent of direct sales in the U.S., according to the latest stats available (2021) from the Direct Selling Association (DSA), an MLM trade group.[32] That percentage has been increasing more or less consistently for at least a decade, but the growth curve started to go from a modest upward slope to almost a forty-five-degree angle around 2010–2011—coinciding with the rise of social media and the explosion of the wellness trend. Why are there so many MLMs in the wellness space? "In short, there is A LOT of money to be made," says William Keep, a professor of marketing at The College of New Jersey who studies MLMs and has served as an expert witness in the prosecution of pyramid schemes. He says that's partly because health and wellness is a large and growing industry, with almost no FDA regulation of the products themselves or the claims manufacturers can make about them. Product margins in this sector (the selling price of products minus the cost of making them) are also high, which likely leads to higher profits for manufacturers. Additionally, the value of these products can be hard to prove, making it tough for consumers to compare one product to another—and when comparisons are difficult, that typically leads to higher prices and higher profits. But those profits are heavily concentrated at the top—primarily at the corporate level, and to a lesser extent among the top 1 percent or so of distributors.

MLM distributors are overwhelmingly women—75 percent, according to the DSA. MLMs have targeted women since their inception: Amway, the originator of the MLM model, got its start selling dietary supplements and home-care products to 1950s housewives. (Today, Amway is a multibillion-dollar business with a lot of political sway: it was cofounded by Richard DeVos Sr., the father-in-law of former Republican Party operative and Trump-era secretary of education Betsy DeVos, and it gives millions in contributions to GOP candidates.) Women who don't or can't work outside the home because of childcare duties are often vulnerable to MLM recruitment, with its promises of being a "mompreneur" and "girlboss" supporting your family while working part-time from home. The reality for most of these women—having to hustle so much to earn money (or simply break even) that they're stuck posting about their wares on social media night and day, being pulled away from their families in mind if not in body—is far less rosy.

MLMs don't only recruit women as distributors; they also tend to target people who are struggling in some way. Máire O Sullivan, a lecturer in marketing at Ireland's Munster Technological University who studies MLMs, explains that people who end up falling prey to them are often in flux—new moms, recent high school and college graduates, immigrants living far from home and family. Herbalife is known to recruit heavily among Latino immigrants, who need income and may not have the connections or language skills to get jobs easily—or may be undocumented and therefore unlikely to denounce the company when they almost inevitably lose money, for fear of drawing attention to their status. Health issues, financial troubles, and relationship problems can also make people vulnerable to MLM recruitment. People in these situations are often feeling adrift and looking for connection, meaning, and success in their lives, and MLMs are right there to sell it to them.

It's a powerful pitch, as Roberta Blevins knows well. In 2014, Blevins had a toddler at home and was struggling with depression, having recently lost her father to pancreatic cancer. She'd gained some weight due to the stress of the loss and the coping method she'd developed to handle it: secretly eating fast food in her car, in order to hide it from her fat-shaming then husband.

When her cousin, whom she describes as one of her favorite people, started selling weight-loss products with a then-obscure MLM called ItWorks!, Blevins got hooked. Here was someone whom she trusted implicitly, offering her a magic bullet that would supposedly shrink her body and make her feel like her old self again. But the ItWorks! products didn't work for her—at least not in the long run, though the "after" photos she shot in the morning while standing up as straight as possible and sucking in her stomach created the illusion that she'd lost weight. Both Blevins and her cousin have since left the MLM world and now see these companies as "a giant scam," says Blevins, who has become a vocal critic of MLMs after her experience selling leggings with another (famously bad) one: LuLaRoe.

The fact that Gary Young started getting serious about the MLM business model around the time he moved to Utah is probably no coincidence. For one thing, he had gotten remarried, and his new wife, Mary, had previously been involved with another MLM and claimed to have had tremendous success. What's more, as *Insider* reported, Young may have realized that the MLM model of using independent contractors to sell products through word of mouth and informal channels "could be his golden ticket to becoming the alternative-health guru he always yearned to become, without having to constantly butt heads with the law." Having people who weren't his employees sell his products and disseminate his message would be a way to avoid being accused of practicing medicine without a license (even though in some sense he was still doing precisely that). If the move was intentional, it worked: Young wasn't arrested again. And the MLM model has been a boon from a financial perspective: Young Living was worth $1.5 billion as of 2020.

Today, Young Living is one of hundreds of wellness companies using an MLM structure. Distributors sell and recruit heavily on social media for wellness-related MLMs like Young Living, dōTERRA (another essential-oil company that was founded in

2008 by a group that included three former Young Living executives), Herbalife, ItWorks!, BeachBody, Isagenix, Juice Plus+, Nu Skin, Optavia, Plexus, Arbonne, and many others, both in public posts touting the supposed benefits of the products, and in private messages to people in their networks. The approach used in those messages is almost inevitably the same: it starts with a cheery greeting ("hey hun!") from a friend, someone you went to high school with, or maybe even someone you barely know, who then moves on to pitching you on their product or "business opportunity." That technique has spawned its own slang in anti-MLM circles: getting put in the "hun zone." Anyone who's experienced it knows the chilling effect that "hun zoning" often has on friendships.

Young passed away in 2018, and the company claims to have evolved past its roots, not wanting to be held responsible for the sins of its father. Although Young still seems to have rock-star status within the company, today Young Living is run by Mary Young. As the company told *Insider* in a statement upon reading the magazine's in-depth, investigative piece about Gary Young, "These allegations simply do not reflect the company that Young Living has evolved to be today, instead referring to events that happened years (and even decades) ago to provide an inaccurate and sensationalized view of Young Living." Of course companies can and do change and evolve throughout the course of their existence. And some people swear by Young Living's products for helping manage all kinds of different symptoms, even if there isn't science to support their claims.

But there are some things about the nature of the company—and of all MLMs—that make it hard to trust that they're not just selling you snake oil.

One of the biggest red flags is the way in which the structure of MLMs allows bogus health claims to proliferate. Because MLMs are sold by a dispersed network of independent distributors, the companies aren't able to adequately control marketing claims made by those distributors. There are more than 2.4 million wellness-MLM salespeople in the U.S. alone, according to the DSA's numbers. Those distributors generally aren't trained as health professionals, and yet "whoever signs an agreement with a company such as Amway (Nutrilite products), Herbalife, Nikken, ProHealth, Usana, Tahitian Noni, or Vemma becomes a 'health advisor,'" write MLM researchers Claudia Gross and Dirk Vriens.[33] And those "health advisors" can make some pretty wild claims, even though official corporate guidance tells them not to. Young Living and dōTERRA distributors have claimed their products can cure numerous conditions including herpes, Alzheimer's disease, and cancer. Young Living's website used to claim that cinnamon bark and oregano could prevent the Ebola virus.[34]

Then there's the *Essential Oils Desk Reference*, a 640-page book written by Gary Young and a coauthor, which claims without evidence that various essential oils are effective at treating almost every known disease. Young Living distributors used the *Desk Reference* for many years to promote their products, until the company began officially discouraging the book's use after the FDA sent a warning letter in 2014 citing distributors' claims that essential oils could treat myriad diseases including viral infections, Parkinson's disease, autism, diabetes, and many others. Young's coauthor and another former Young Living employee told *Insider* that in many cases there was no real evidence at all behind the book's claims — they were based on Young's opinions, which he believed were an inspiration from God and were true even if there was no science to support them.[35]

*The New Yorker* reported that in 2017, a dōTERRA distributor answered a question from an attendee at an in-person "Essential Oils 101" class who asked if oils could provide a "natural" solution to keep her sister-in-law's cancer from recurring, as opposed to the pill she was taking that had nasty side effects. "There is an oil for that," the distributor said cautiously. "There is some research. It is an option. It would not have those side effects."[36]

For the record, there actually isn't "an oil for that"—the research she's referring to doesn't support prescribing essential oils to human cancer patients. Although some early-stage research in animal and human cell cultures does show that some essential oils may help prevent cancer cells from proliferating in a petri dish (in vitro studies), that research isn't intended to guide any clinical decisions. You can't study the functioning of cells in a lab or in animals—or in computer models, known as *in silico* studies—and expect the findings to translate to real, live humans. While those types of studies can be important as early litmus tests to determine whether future research is warranted, their results often aren't reproducible in humans. There are just too many differences between those laboratory/computer models and the real, unique, hyper-networked universe that is the human body. To study how things work in that setting, you need to actually *study human bodies* (*in vivo* studies in humans, as opposed to in animals). So in order to find out whether or not essential oils are effective at fighting cancer in humans, you can't just put the oils on cancer cells in a lab and see what happens. That's a start, but then you'd need to conduct human *in vivo* trials that are randomized, controlled, and double-blind—the only study design that can tell if a treatment is truly effective and not merely the result of placebo effects. And you'd need large enough studies and multiple studies by different groups of scientists using that design, because in order for research to be reliable it has to be replicable.

The existing studies on essential oils and cancer (and on essential oils and most diseases, for that matter) simply don't meet the criteria for evidence-based medicine. They're preliminary investigations that say things like "[XYZ] essential oil can be regarded as a candidate for *in vivo* studies"[37] and "future pre-clinical and clinical studies are urgently needed to evaluate the safety and efficacy of [ABC] essential oil as a therapeutic agent for treating cancer."[38] These early-stage studies have proliferated in recent years—the literature on essential oils and cancer has seen exponential growth since 2009, according to PubMed—and there are now thousands of papers investigating the potential use of different essential oils for various types of cancer and other diseases. Still, as science goes, this literature is in its infancy. These studies can't be taken as anything more than an interesting guide for future research.

Meanwhile, the science on COVID-19 is in what might be described as its embryonic stage—and yet wellness MLM distributors have made wild claims about how their products supposedly prevent and cure COVID. "If interested to learn more or obtain oils or rollers Let me know," a dōTERRA rep wrote on social media in 2020. "A little extra protection can help #doterra #NursesCOVID19 #Dialysis #ImmunityBoosters #ImproveRespiratoryFunction." Or as a distributor for Isagenix posted without evidence, "In the fight against COVID-19—Keep moving every day and eating healthy! Isagenix shakes boost your immunity 500%!" In 2020, the FTC sent warning letters to at least sixteen wellness MLMs for their distributors' false health claims—and/or false earnings claims, which were also common during the pandemic, as MLM reps tried to capitalize on the economic crisis to recruit more people for their downline. As a distributor for the skin care MLM Arbonne wrote on social media, "Living in quarantine and where 14 million people applied for unemployment just last week...I'll stick with the opportunity to change people's lives...turn a small investment into six figures....#arbonne...#quarantine #2020."[39]

O Sullivan says that in general, most MLM companies have rules about what health claims and financial promises distributors are allowed to make. "Most of them have clear guidelines; whether they enforce them downstream, that seems to be more up for grabs." This guidance often takes the form of "say this, not that" documents that outline what is and isn't allowed. But because of the DSHEA law that we discussed in Chapter 2, supplement companies are still allowed to make structure-function claims—which leaves a lot of room to *imply* that their products prevent disease and keep you in an optimal state of wellness. For example, according to a 2015 Young Living guidance document, reps can say things like "maintains healthy lung function" but not "maintains healthy lungs in smokers," or "supports kidney health and function" but not "cures kidney infection," or "can be used as a part of your healthy diet to help maintain a healthy blood sugar level" but not "use as a part of your diet when taking insulin to help maintain healthy blood sugar levels." To the average reader, is there really much difference between these claims? I'm a licensed healthcare provider with a master's degree in public health, and I found the Young Living guidance document somewhat unclear. Why should typical distributors with little to no health-related education be expected to make sense of it?

Young Living told *Insider* in 2020 that in recent years, the company "has doubled down on its compliance program to educate and police its members to ensure that accurate and proven claims about its products are being made." It said that it "promotes only FDA-compliant marketing material and all members are instructed to only use materials approved by Young Living." But the very fact that MLMs don't—and really can't—vet all their reps' communications *before* they're posted online makes even the most robust compliance program something like a game of whack-a-mole, where they have to go around striking down false claims after they've popped up. They can't possibly have enough resources to catch every instance of misinformation their distributors post—and even if they did, untold numbers of people would already have been exposed to it by the time it got taken down. Much like the anti-vax misinformation that was allowed to proliferate on Facebook and other social media platforms before being removed in a scattershot way late in the pandemic, false health claims by MLM distributors get seen, shared, and reshared enough to do significant damage, even if they're ultimately deleted. It's also hard to ignore another parallel with social media companies' handling of anti-vax misinformation: MLMs may have a financial incentive *not* to remove misleading health claims, since those claims often help sell product.

I asked O Sullivan if she thinks MLM companies are deliberately looking the other way when it comes to their distributors' marketing language. "I won't say that," she says. "But I have to say, I see an awful lot of [false claims], and I don't see an awful lot of cracking down." When there are egregious assertions being made about products, like the COVID-19 claims, federal agencies might step in—but it doesn't necessarily do much to change things in the long run. "It seems to me that people get a rap on the knuckles," she says, which might temporarily stop distributors from making those claims online. But they may still be making them—just not in writing, and/or not in public forums. Indeed, some former MLM distributors have shared that although they're officially discouraged from posting health claims publicly, it's a different story in direct messages, private Facebook groups, and house parties, where health claims often flow liberally. "I think that there certainly is a lot more room for enforcement," O Sullivan says. "If you say something bad about an MLM, there's plenty of lawyers who will track you down. So I don't know why if you say something outrageously good, like 'we cure cancer,' there's not a team there to crack down on that."

## Workplace Unwellness

In 2009, Steven Burd, then CEO of the Safeway grocery chain, launched a PR campaign to promote his company's workplace-wellness plan, which was among the first wave of such programs. Safeway's program was launched in 2005, Burd claimed, to "reward healthy behavior" among its employees by giving them discounts for passing tests related to tobacco usage, weight, blood pressure, and cholesterol levels. As he wrote in an op-ed for the *Wall Street Journal,* during the four-year period since the program's launch, the company apparently kept its per-capita healthcare costs the same, whereas most American companies' costs increased by nearly 40 percent in the same time frame.[40] "By our calculation, if the nation had adopted our approach in 2005, the nation's direct health-care bill would be $550 billion less than it is today," Burd wrote.

His ultimate argument was that *increasing* financial rewards for employees' "healthy behavior" would save even more in healthcare costs, yet existing legislation was standing in the way. Under the then-current regulations, incentives for meeting wellness goals were limited to 20 percent of the insurance premium. "Today, we are constrained by current laws from increasing these incentives," he wrote. "If these limits are appropriately increased, I am confident Safeway's per capita health-care costs will decline for at least another five years as our work force becomes healthier."

At a time when the battle over American healthcare reform was at its peak, policy makers on both sides of the aisle were persuaded by Burd's claims.

There was one problem with his story: Almost none of it was true.

As *Washington Post* reporter David Hilzenrath discovered by reviewing company documents and interviewing senior staff, while Safeway's healthcare costs did remain more or less flat between 2005 and 2009, it had nothing to do with the company's program of "rewarding healthy behaviors."[41] In fact, Safeway had only implemented its workplace-wellness program in 2009, mere months—not years—before Burd's op-ed was published. What's more, only about 14 percent of the company's workforce (the non-union workers) was even eligible to participate in the program—not nearly enough to sway costs so significantly. Instead, Safeway's healthcare savings came from a 2006 decision to raise deductibles and shift more costs onto employees.

By the time Hilzenrath broke that story in January of 2010, however, it was too late. Politicians in charge of healthcare reform had already bought Burd's specious story—and it fundamentally reshaped the healthcare landscape in the U.S. "The Safeway program has proven so successful that the company wants to increase its incentives for rewarding healthy behavior," Republican senator Mitch McConnell said in a 2009 speech on the Senate floor. "Unfortunately, current laws restrict it from doing so."[42] President Obama also repeatedly touted Safeway's supposed successes with workplace wellness, even after Burd's falsehoods came to light. "It's a program that has helped Safeway cut health-care spending by 13 percent and workers save over 20 percent on their premiums," he told the American Medical Association in a June 2010 speech.[43] When Obama delivered those remarks, Safeway's program was less than six months old—and its spending was actually on the rise, according to the company's own analysis.

Despite being based on a lie, with so much bipartisan support, the so-called Safeway Amendment soon was incorporated into the Affordable Care Act of 2010. From there, workplace-wellness programs spread like wildfire, becoming a booming industry whose revenue more than tripled between 2010 and 2018.[44] More than 50 million American workers take part in these programs, often without much of a choice—in many cases they're mandatory if you want employer-based health insurance.[45] A 2021 report by the Kaiser Family Foundation found that 83 percent of large companies (with two hundred or more employees) and 58 percent of smaller firms offer a workplace wellness program of some kind.[46] Globally, the market for workplace wellness was valued at nearly $50 billion in 2019 and is projected to be worth roughly $66.2 billion by 2027.[47]

Though the Safeway con that kicked off the workplace-wellness trend may be somewhat anomalous, the industry as a whole is incredibly problematic in its own right. Indeed, it's starting to seem more and more like one massive rip-off that's taking advantage of employers and harming employees while enriching the industry. To be sure, it's a different breed of scheme than Gibson's false claims of "naturally" curing her cancer or MLMs' unsubstantiated assertions that their products can prevent and cure disease (and that people can make money selling them). Workplace wellness has a higher veneer of respectability than someone touting essential oils as a COVID cure; to many people these workplace programs sound "sensible" and unlikely to cause harm. But one thing workplace wellness shares with these scams is deceptiveness—it promises one thing and delivers something very different. And evidence is mounting that not only do workplace wellness programs fail to lower costs for employers as advertised, but they also don't actually work for promoting well-being.

Take a 2019 randomized controlled trial (RCT), in which researchers designed and implemented a workplace-wellness program for a large employer (the University of Illinois at Urbana-Champaign).[48] The program was quite comprehensive (and typical of many such programs), with an annual on-site biometric health screening, an annual online health-risk assessment, and weekly wellness activities. Previous research on workplace-wellness programs tended to be plagued by self-selection bias (employees who already engage in more wellness behaviors tend to be more likely to sign up for workplace-wellness programs in the first place). To try to minimize the effects of that bias, the researchers randomly assigned 3,300 study subjects to a "treatment group" that received paid time off to participate in the wellness program, and assigned another 1,534 subjects to a control group, which was not allowed to participate. Members of the treatment group who completed the entire two-year program were randomly assigned to receive rewards valued between $50 and $650.

Despite strong participation, the researchers didn't find that the workplace-wellness program had *any* significant effect on forty out of forty-two outcomes studied, including various measures of medical spending, productivity, health behaviors, and self-reported health. The program had only two effects that were statistically significant, if underwhelming: people in the treatment group were more likely than those in the control group to report ever having received a health screening; and those in the treatment group were more likely to say that "management prioritizes worker health and safety"—but only during the first year. All in all, the program was a real bust.

The study, however, was quite important, being one of the first-ever RCTs in the workplace-wellness field. Because of its randomized design, the researchers were able to compare their results to the existing scientific literature and found that their estimates could refute most of the previous findings on medical spending and absenteeism reported in 112 prior studies.

As it happened, another, much larger RCT conducted at the same time by a different group of researchers produced much the same results. That study was done by researchers from the University of Chicago and Harvard, this time among employees at BJ's Wholesale Club.[49] The scientists randomly assigned 20 BJ's stores to offer a wellness program to all their employees, and then compared the outcomes with those at 140 stores that didn't offer the program. In all, nearly 33,000 workers from 160 BJ's outlets were involved in the study, including a diverse workforce and a substantial number of lower-income employees. On offer was a series of four- to eight-week modules covering key wellness topics—including nutrition, physical activity, stress reduction, and prevention—taught by registered dietitians, as well as a personal health assessment survey and biometric screening. The program was administered by a well-established workplace-wellness company.

After eighteen months, worksites that participated in the

wellness program had two statistically significant results: more employees reported engaging in regular exercise and actively managing their weight. But there were no significant differences in other behaviors (such as smoking, alcohol use, sleep, or fruit and vegetable consumption) or in self-reported health (including measures of mental health). What's more, there were no significant differences in *clinical* markers of health, like cholesterol, blood pressure, and blood sugar. There was also no difference in employees' BMI between the participating and nonparticipating worksites, despite the fact that more wellness-program participants were *trying* to manage their weight. Finally, the two groups didn't differ in terms of healthcare spending or utilization, or productivity measures like absenteeism or job performance. The researchers then followed up with both groups in a 2021 study to see if anything had changed three years after the program— and the only thing that had is that the percentages of people engaging in regular physical activity and weight management had both declined by several points.[50]

Not only do workplace-wellness programs not "work" in the sense of creating the changes they're intended to create, but they're also often harmful to well-being. For starters they're massively ableist, forcing people with certain health conditions to pay higher premiums and incentivizing (some say coercing) employees to give up sensitive data like genetic information and family medical histories, which also can be used to justify premium hikes. The Americans with Disabilities Act of 1990 (ADA) and the Genetic Information Nondiscrimination Act (GINA) of 2008 theoretically should prevent such discrimination, but the Equal Employment Opportunity Commission (EEOC) carved out exceptions to those laws for corporate wellness programs, issuing guidance that allowed employers to offer insurance-premium discounts of as much as 30 percent to workers who joined the programs. A 2017 lawsuit forced the EEOC to retract this guidance, successfully arguing that the 30 percent rule allowed companies to unfairly penalize employees for opting out of wellness programs, in violation of the ADA and GINA. But as of this writing, the EEOC has not said when it plans to propose new rules or guidance for workplace-wellness programs, and programs continue to offer "incentives" for joining, effectively fining workers for not taking part. Meanwhile, millions of people who are already stigmatized in wellness culture — like those with diabetes, heart disease, or a high BMI — have legally been charged thousands of dollars more for insurance than their coworkers.

Carrie Dennett, a journalist and registered dietitian, is intimately familiar with the harm these programs cause, having worked as a copywriter for nearly ten years at a company that produced health and wellness programs for corporations and insurance companies. In 2010, around the time that her company began rolling out workplace-wellness programs for its clients, it also implemented annual weight-loss and fitness challenges for its own employees. These challenges involved competing to beat coworkers in categories like percentage of weight lost, pedometer steps, and exercise minutes. At the time, Dennett was already a hard-core dieter and was participating in an online "fat-burning" program, but the workplace challenge took her dieting to a whole new level. She started exercising compulsively. "If I got less than about [X] steps a day, I felt like I was a total loser," she says. She won both of the exercise challenges she entered, but her behavior became very disordered in the process, though it never tipped over into a full-blown eating disorder. "If I was predisposed to developing an eating disorder, that probably would have done it," she says. In retrospect, she's pretty sure one of her colleagues (and primary competitors in the challenge) was already struggling with a restrictive eating disorder.

I've worked with numerous clients in recovery from eating disorders and subclinical disordered eating who dread the regular weigh-ins, nutrition challenges, and biometric measurements that take place at their companies, often feeling triggered back into disordered behaviors by the onslaught of diet culture in the workplace. Yet they feel like they have no choice but to participate in these programs, because otherwise they have to pay hundreds or sometimes thousands of dollars more in insurance premiums each year. And bringing a healthcare provider's note to exempt them from participation often doesn't keep them from getting penalized.

Even if participation in certain workplace-wellness activities is truly optional, like the "lunch and learn" workshops put on by some companies, the unintended consequences for people with disordered eating are very real. "During my own tenure at a wellness company, while I was dealing with the vestiges of anorexia, the leadership team invited a specialist to our office to talk about the benefits of intermittent fasting," a writer named Charlotte Lieberman shared in a 2019 piece for *Harvard Business Review*.[51] "Although I was no longer restricting calories, I was fixated on regaining my discipline, and constantly blamed myself for 'giving in' to my hunger. As I listened to the speaker, I felt shame. My deepest insecurities were validated, and I starved myself the rest of the day."

Even if workplace-wellness programs pay lip service to mental health, they generally aren't helpful—and can often be harmful—to those who are struggling with genuine mental-health issues. They look at surface-level behaviors like exercise or eating habits without examining the motivations behind them—and without measuring the unintended psychological impacts of being financially coerced into engaging in those behaviors. These programs prioritize these behaviors, as well as physical characteristics like weight or blood-pressure levels, above true well-being. "The only job I've ever had that promoted wellness treated me the worst when I was at my least well," a former chef at a popular retreat center told Lieberman. The company had employee perks like free gym access, discounted spa treatments, and sessions with a nutritionist, but no mental-health leave whatsoever. When the chef had to be hospitalized for three weeks because of her bipolar disorder, she was fired for missing too many days at work.

If workplace-wellness programs don't actually produce lasting wellness, what's the point of them? Likely to make their creators money. Dennett says that when she worked at the workplace-wellness company, they seemed fixated on showing their clients the "ROI" (return on investment) they could get by signing up. But it wasn't always easy. "There didn't appear to be an ROI, because I know there was a pretty high amount of client turnover," Dennett says. "Clients wouldn't be seeing an ROI at the end of their contract with my company, so they would end the contract, and either not pursue another workplace wellness program or go on to the next company that offered one, thinking maybe theirs is better. That tells me that it wasn't working in the sense it was designed to work." Her experience in her own workplace confirmed that for the vast majority, these programs don't create lasting well-being. "Honestly, among my fellow employees, I didn't see that anybody was better off for it," she says. "I really see no benefit whatsoever for workplace wellness programs because they just don't promote wellness, and that's really the bottom line."

The same could be said for other aspects of wellness culture, from multilevel marketing to assorted forms of snake oil and outright lies from influencers capitalizing on false claims. The abundance of predatory practices makes us vulnerable, and the failures of institutions that should be taking care of us increases our vulnerability. Although restoring public confidence is a tall order in the current landscape for many reasons, one important thing institutions could do to earn back trust is to implement regulations (and enforce existing ones) that would help safeguard us from wellness culture and promote true well-being. We'll turn to some of those potential policy changes next.

# CHAPTER 8

# From Wellness to Well-Being

The idea that life is best spent in an endless quest to achieve "optimized" health—or to eradicate existing chronic illnesses through some mythically perfect, "natural" approach that isn't actually supported by sound evidence—often leads to mental strife and greater stress, and sometimes even to more physical-health issues. The mind-body connection is strong, and stress is a well-documented risk factor for a whole host of physical ailments. The disordered eating promoted by wellness culture also can lead directly to problems with digestion and other body systems, triggering and exacerbating chronic conditions, as it did for many of the people we met in previous chapters. Prioritizing physical health can come at the expense of other aspects of life—career, relationships, finances, community—or can become a poor substitute for them. And for many people it's difficult to dabble in wellness culture without getting sucked in to a degree that compromises our overall well-being. It might start with something like acupuncture for pain management that then leads to other alternative providers and practices. These may eventually lead to an obsession with eating "clean" and getting off all conventional medications. The mental and emotional ramifications of going down such a path are routinely ignored in the supposedly "holistic" domains of complementary, integrative, and functional medicine. Moreover, powerful algorithms that detect an interest in wellness topics can serve us increasingly extreme content, leading us down rabbit holes of disinformation that ultimately threaten the well-being of entire communities.

Instead of wellness, which in practice is mostly about physical health, what I think many of us are really after is *well-being*, a truly holistic measure of our mental, emotional, social, and economic condition. Well-being encompasses overall life satisfaction and satisfaction in specific areas of life, as well as a sense of purpose, autonomy, and agency. It encompasses social determinants of health like feeling safe in your community and having stable employment. Well-being doesn't require physical perfection or constant optimization. It doesn't necessitate being entirely symptom-free or medication-free. It's possible to be in a state of relative well-being even while living with chronic conditions, which are typically painted as barriers to wellness.

Wellness culture is a trap, keeping us stuck in a narrow view of what it means to be well and exposing us to much that is harmful—weight stigma, scams, conspiracy theories, damaging approaches to mental health, false diagnoses. To break free from that trap and find our way to true well-being—whatever that might look like for each of us—we can learn to be discerning about the information we consume and engage in practices that support us mentally and emotionally, not just physically. There are ways to help navigate wellness culture without getting ensnared in it, as we'll discuss. But working on individual behavior is not enough. Not everyone has the capacity to make major changes on their own, and social problems aren't really individual responsibilities anyway. We need change at the cultural, institutional, and policy levels to help undo the harm caused by wellness culture and create a society that truly supports well-being for everyone. Solutions to the many problems that wellness culture presents have to be systemic and collective, not simply personal and private. Social change is the most pressing. And while specific policy change to improve well-being in various

237

communities goes beyond the scope of this book, here are a few broad approaches that could make a world of difference.

## Societal Approaches

*End Healthism and Address Social Determinants*

It's natural for people to want health and wellness for themselves and their loved ones, and yet the single-minded pursuit of these goals can have deeply negative consequences, as we've seen. In fact, most of the problems inherent in wellness culture stem from underlying healthism—the pervasive Western belief that health is a supreme moral value, the primary measure of well-being, and a matter of individual (rather than collective) responsibility, located solely in the body of the patient.

Political economist Robert Crawford coined the term *healthism* in 1980, after witnessing an explosion in the "holistic health" movement—the forerunner of what I'm now calling wellness culture, and especially its complementary and alternative medicine component. In his seminal paper "Healthism and the Medicalization of Everyday Life," Crawford points out that although the holistic-health movement claimed to be about treating the whole person—including emotional, mental, and spiritual aspects—in reality it still viewed health and disease as properties of the individual mind and body, with solutions based on personal lifestyle choices.[1]

He cites a passage from a 1978 holistic-health handbook that sounds like it would be right at home on an Instagram wellness influencer's page today, in which the author warns against the "negativity" of attributing health problems to the outer environment and writes that "health and happiness *can* be ours if we desire; we can create our personal reality, down to the finest detail." Another 1970s holistic-health tome illustrates the flip side of belief in such a high level of personal responsibility: "We choose our sickness when, through neglect or ignorance, we allow it to spread within us.... We should not fool ourselves into thinking that disease is caused by an enemy from without. We are responsible for our disease."[2] In other words, if we are sick, we have only ourselves to blame.

In these ways, the holistic-health movement remained (and remains) mired in the neoliberal worldview that plagues the entire health and wellness industry. That worldview conceives of health as the responsibility of the individual, blames people for their own health challenges, and essentially ignores social conditions and their impact on well-being.

Instead of staying attached to wellness culture's individualistic approach to health, we need to address the social determinants of health at the systemic level, including in public health programs and in healthcare. The social determinants might ostensibly center around "health," but in fact they address well-being because they encompass the whole person and the communities in which we live. More important, they don't individualize problems, and they take into account social conditions at every step of the way.

Attending to social determinants means implementing policies to end poverty and increasing access to quality care. This might include, in the U.S., adding a robust public option, or instituting universal healthcare; in other countries, it might require significantly increasing government investment in public healthcare systems. It will inevitably involve rooting out the racism, misogyny, anti-fat bias, ableism, and other forms of prejudice in health-related institutions that harm people and make them lose faith in conventional medicine. Over time, these changes could help lead to better care for people who were previously failed by the healthcare system, which may help instill trust in that system—and in turn may help keep people from falling prey to damaging wellness trends.

*Foreground Mental Well-Being*

As I write this, I'm nine months postpartum. During my pregnancy I went to the obstetrician's office every few weeks (every week by the end), and at none of those visits did my doctors ask about my mental health. There was always discussion of how I was feeling physically, time to ask questions about anything going on in my body, and a check on uterine growth and the baby's heart to make sure she was developing well. I did feel that my physical health was taken seriously in this system. But no one ever asked how I was *feeling* about the pregnancy, or how my relationship with food and my body was going—even though the providers knew my history of disordered eating, anxiety, and PTSD. After giving birth, at my two-week and six-week checkups, I got those rote questionnaires that asked, essentially, "in the past 7 days, have you felt sad, depressed, or anxious, or had difficulty coping?"—which was something, though definitely not enough. I'd had a traumatic birth experience and struggled with an extended version of the postpartum blues, and I answered "sometimes" to many of the questions, but none of the doctors or nurses I saw ever brought it up.

Granted, maybe that was because I didn't meet the criteria for postpartum depression, and they were saving their limited time for patients who did. But it's also likely that they just didn't feel equipped to talk about mental-health concerns. Unless they go on to specialize in psychiatry, medical doctors generally aren't trained in mental health—a systemic issue that goes far beyond these individual providers—and untrained practitioners who wade into the realm of psychology can undoubtedly do harm. (Likewise, in alternative-health spaces, ideas such as repressed memories and manifesting can spread and cause significant damage.) It's understandable that most medical school programs wouldn't spend much time on mental health, given the amount of physical-health content that has to be covered, but it leaves physicians poorly equipped to deal with the realities and complexities of their patients' lives.

In 2017, the Des Moines University medical school, a top producer of primary care physicians, announced plans to implement a three-day, fifteen-hour course on mental health developed by the National Alliance on Mental Illness for all third-year students. The *Des Moines Register* called the plan "groundbreaking."[3] Surely the program, which has been going since 2018, has helped many students develop greater awareness of mental-health issues—yet the fact that even such a short training is so rare and revolutionary in medical schools indicates how far the field still has to go in making mental health a priority.

The same is true in public health. "Even though public health has made a lot of advances as a field in recognizing the power and importance of mental health, still I think we tend to not prioritize it or weigh the impacts of mental health as much as we should," U.S. surgeon general Vivek Murthy said in a 2021 podcast interview.[4] "Mental health is part of our overall health, and we have to treat it that way."

To that end, medical schools and public health programs need to do more to train future doctors and public health professionals. A three-hour course is a start, but discussion of mental and emotional well-being really should be woven into every med-school curriculum and every public health program. I'm not talking about medical models of mental health, which tend to reduce all mental and emotional issues to chemical imbalances in the brain, correctable with drugs, but really about attending to patients' and clients' overall well-being. Treating and preventing physical-health ailments certainly is important and is a priority for many patients, but that shouldn't come at the expense of mental health, as it too often does now. If overall well-being is harmed in the pursuit of physical health, then is there even a net benefit? Or have providers just created new problems that they're not equipped to solve?

*Regulate Big Tech*

Whistleblower Frances Haugen revealed her identity and testified before Congress in October 2021. Haugen, a former Facebook employee, had already released tens of thousands of pages of the company's internal research and documents, which became the basis for the *Wall Street Journal*'s influential investigative-reporting series "The Facebook Files," and, later, numerous other media reports. At her first congressional hearing, Haugen testified that Facebook's products "harm children, stoke division, and weaken our democracy," putting their astronomical profits before people and moral responsibility.[5] She called on Congress to regulate Facebook and other social media companies through legislative measures, including amending Section 230 of the Communications Decency Act—which, as discussed in Chapters 4 and 5, absolves social media platforms of legal responsibility for content their users post, even if that content is anti-vaccine misinformation, health conspiracy theories, or other similarly harmful material.

As I write this, it's been more than a year since Haugen initially came forward, and there are now nearly a dozen bills before Congress (and many more discussion drafts) attempting to address the numerous problems with social media and Big Tech in general that she and others have pointed out. Several more congressional hearings on tech issues have been held since, notably without the presence of the executives who used to be fixtures at such events, including Mark Zuckerberg (who drew particular ire from representatives for lying in previous congressional testimony). Hearings have addressed how social platforms facilitate the spread of misinformation and violence, target children, enable illegal drug sales, undermine democracy, promote discrimination, and threaten privacy and national security. Predictably, there are different focuses on the two sides of the aisle, with Republicans focusing more on national security, illegal activity, and perceived censorship of conservative views, and Democrats focusing more on mis- and disinformation, violence, discrimination, and undermining democracy.

Still, bipartisan interest in some sort of regulation is strong, particularly with regard to how technology impacts kids.

The details of how to accomplish such regulation are nuanced, and I certainly don't have all the answers. But I do know that we desperately need to regulate social media and other user-generated-content platforms. We must create a better social media environment that doesn't amplify toxic wellness messages at every turn. Instead, social media platforms should help slow the spread of conspiracy theories and encourage people to think critically about what they're reading. To that end, there are some policy proposals that seem promising:

First, we could make tech companies accountable for harmful misinformation amplified by their algorithms, because in influencing what gets viewed and shared these companies are acting like publishers. Newspapers, magazines, TV and radio shows, and other traditional media are legally prohibited from knowingly spreading false information, and they can be held liable for any violations. Because of this potential liability, these outlets typically perform fact-checking and vetting of their content, ensuring that patently false claims — like much of the wellness misinformation and anti-vax content that gets spread on social media — aren't published. The system isn't perfect, as spreaders of misinformation often avoid legal accountability by using the defense that they were merely expressing an opinion — or that they were engaging in exaggeration that shouldn't be taken literally, as lawyers for Tucker Carlson of *Fox News* successfully argued in a 2020 slander suit.[6] Still, people at least have the opportunity to mount a legal case against traditional media companies for spreading falsehoods. For those who've been harmed by mis- and disinformation spread through social media algorithms, there's no such recourse, because tech platforms are essentially shielded from all liability under Section 230.

Congress should remove these blanket legal protections and

require tech platforms to abide by a "duty of care" to their users. As numerous tech-reform experts have noted, the people who build everything from roads to buildings to kitchen appliances are already bound by such a duty. "I have to do more safety testing and go through more compliance procedures to create a toaster than to create Facebook," Cambridge Analytica whistleblower Christopher Wylie told the BBC in 2020.[7] Why shouldn't social media companies be equally responsible for their products? Regulators could require them to catalog all the harms and potential harms their platforms might cause, go through testing and quality control, and be responsible for unintended consequences.

This is particularly important when it comes to algorithms that prioritize engagement, because such algorithms have a demonstrated history of causing harm. As Haugen told a Senate panel in 2021, algorithms shouldn't be protected by Section 230.[8] She advocates making a distinction between content posted by users and content amplified by algorithms, and holding tech companies liable for content only when their algorithms boost it. This would effectively help quarantine misinformation and keep it from spreading virally as it does now, while still allowing users to post freely.

Critics of tech reform often invoke freedom of speech when arguing that the platforms shouldn't be subject to government regulation, but that's a bit of a red herring. Though it's important to look at the potential impact of any Internet regulation on freedom of speech and expression, the online environment is very different from the town square. Just because you're legally free to say something doesn't mean tech companies owe you a megaphone—freedom of speech doesn't mean freedom of reach, as the saying goes. "There is no right to algorithmic amplification," Renée DiResta, the information-technology researcher we met in Chapter 5, wrote in 2018.[9] For one thing, social media platforms are private organizations with their own terms of service (TOS) that they're able to enforce as they see fit. But TOS aside, people are at liberty to say whatever they want on social media, just as they could in a real-life public square. They can spout health misinformation or any other false claims until they're blue in the face—but they don't have a constitutional right to get their words broadcast to thousands or millions of people. In the legal sense, freedom of speech essentially just means people can't be prosecuted for speaking their mind (although there are important exceptions, such as the prohibition on using speech to incite violence or chaos, like yelling "fire" in a crowded theater). Reducing the reach of mis- and disinformation doesn't infringe on anyone's freedom of speech.

In addition to being held responsible for algorithmic amplification, tech companies can and should put checks in place to limit the spread of false information on their platforms. There are many ways they can do that: stopping new content from reaching a large audience until after it's fact-checked; limiting the number of times a piece of content can be reshared with just a click (requiring users to copy and paste to share after that limit is reached, which encourages people to stop and think before resharing); preventing known mis- and disinformation from showing up in people's news feeds; and not recommending accounts or groups that consistently promote false information.

It's also essential that tech companies make their algorithms more transparent and just. There are generally two kinds of algorithms that social platforms use: recommendation algorithms and content-moderation algorithms. The recommendation algorithms are what often feeds mis- and disinformation to users, and these algorithms also generally give advertisers the ability to target their campaigns at certain groups, including marginalized groups. For example, anti-vax entrepreneur Robert F. Kennedy Jr. used social media to blast vaccine misinformation out specifically to Black people, according to a December 2021 congressional testimony by Imran Ahmed of the Center for Countering Digital Hate.[10] The second type of algorithm, the content-moderation algorithm, theoretically is supposed to catch and ban such misinformation. But the artificial intelligence (AI) that social platforms use for moderation is woefully inadequate to the task. The supposed proficiency of AI moderation is "one of the big lies that the tech industry has been selling us," Nathalie Maréchal, a researcher and policy manager at Ranking Digital Rights, told Congress in the same hearing. "They want us to believe that they're just around the corner from being able to [...use AI to] identify and moderate away all the direct sales, all the incitement to violence, all the hate speech, all the content that we are rightly concerned about today, [but] that is not true—only human judgment can do that."[11] Tech companies need to be pushed to invest in content moderation by humans—and to make their recommendation algorithms more disinformation-proof in the first place.

Congress also could restrict the types of advertising available on social platforms, in order to take away the financial incentives for platforms to serve up extreme content to vulnerable people. Right now, the platforms' business model is based primarily on surveillance advertising, in which tech companies collect enormous amounts of personal data from users (through both their behavior on the platforms and across the Internet, thanks to cross-site tracking) and use that data to serve targeted ads. This kind of advertising isn't just creepy, it's also deeply harmful. It allows companies to zero in on users' vulnerabilities—for example, people who express an interest in dieting or "healthy eating" getting targeted with dangerous diet products, or new moms getting served anti-vax content. As one group of international tech-reform advocates argued in a 2020 report, lawmakers should require social media companies to tell users *why* specific pieces of content are being recommended to them, and consider limiting the ability to target advertising based on users' private, personal data.[12]

If you live in the U.S. and want to support these reforms, you can call your senators and your House representative to let them know. (As much as many of us abhor the phone, it's still widely considered to be the best way to make your voice heard in Congress.) Visit house.gov and senate.gov for contact info, or call the United States Capitol switchboard at (202) 224-3121 and ask for your congresspeople by name.

*Regulate the Supplement Industry*

Of the societal/policy approaches to addressing wellness culture, this one is probably the least likely to be taken — because of the astronomical amount of lobbying money that's been flowing from the supplement industry to American politicians on both sides of the aisle for decades. But the industry desperately needs regulation.

Specifically, Congress should repeal DSHEA, the 1994 law that barred the FDA from testing or approving herbal and dietary supplements before they hit the market. Supplements are mostly ineffective and useless, but some can have powerful effects (and side effects) as well as unforeseen interactions with other drugs. What's more, there have been many cases in which supplements were found to be adulterated with drugs that weren't listed on the label, causing significant harm to consumers. Herbal and dietary supplements should be regulated in the same way pharmaceutical drugs are, with mandatory premarket testing for safety and efficacy. And advertising for supplements should undergo preapproval and be required to list side effects and risks, as is necessary for drugs.

## Individual Approaches

*Sift through Misinformation*

As an individual there's only so much you can do to navigate the rough waters of wellness culture, but learning how to distinguish between harmful health misinformation and genuinely helpful advice is essential. Developing skills for discernment helps keep you from falling prey to beliefs and behaviors that are likely to worsen your overall well-being. The SIFT check we discussed in the previous chapter is a helpful start. To recap, SIFT stands for

Stop.
Investigate the source.
Find better coverage.
Trace claims, quotes, and media to the original context.

SIFT is designed for quick decision-making about sources of information, which is ideal when you're scrolling through social media or casually consuming online news. But SIFT may not be enough in every situation, and it doesn't address the emotional pull of misinformation. So if you still feel compelled by a particular wellness influencer even after a quick SIFT check, it might help to go deeper. Here are some questions you might ask yourself to help you determine whether a given influencer, product, or practice is credible and helpful, dubious and harmful, or simply ineffective:

Is the source peddling conspiracy theories ("doctors don't want you to get well, they just want to make money") in order to paint itself as the only credible source of wellness information ("we have the secrets to longevity that Big Pharma doesn't want you to know")?

Does learning about or using the product or program expose you to groups or advertisements devoted to other conspiracy theories (anti-vax rhetoric, wild 5G claims, QAnon)?

Is this source using scientific-sounding terms that, upon investigation, don't seem to mean what the source is using them to mean (or don't seem to mean anything at all)? In other words, is it pseudoscience?

Does this source provoke intense emotions in you, but you're not able to verify the facts? Do you experience any physical sensations such as heart racing, sweating, shallow breathing, or tightness in your chest, jaw, or shoulders? Does your nervous system feel activated, or is your mind stuck in a loop of repetitive, self-negating thoughts?

Did you only come across this source after being led there by social media?

Is there credible, robust scientific information—multiple large studies, especially randomized controlled trials in relevant populations, by numerous different groups of researchers without financial ties to the outcomes—to back up any claims about the product or program's effectiveness? Or are these claims based solely on testimonials from individuals?

Is the practice being led by a trusted member of an Indigenous group that you yourself are a part of, in line with long-standing cultural healing traditions? Or in contrast, is the practice part of a culture that you don't belong to, and is it being disseminated by someone who may lack a deep understanding of that culture and its traditions?

Does taking part in this program require you to significantly restrict your eating, invest in multiple expensive supplements, and continue eliminating more and more foods?

If there is testing involved, are the tests wildly expensive? Are they covered by insurance? Do they seem capable of measuring what they purport to measure—or are they simple questionnaires that somehow claim to give an airtight diagnosis?

Does the influencer, product, or program focus exclusively on physical health (even while claiming to address holistic health) and ignore mental health and other important aspects of well-being?

Thinking through these questions may give you a better sense of whether to invest your time, money, and energy in a given wellness product or practice.

*Be a Critical Consumer of Science*

As you sift through information and evaluate sources, you might be tempted to give a pass to any claim that seems to have scientific backing—"trust science," as the political slogan goes. Yet that can actually make you *more* vulnerable to mis- and disinformation, not less. A 2021 study of nearly two thousand people in the U.S. found that having a broad trust in science makes people susceptible to pseudoscience (scientific-sounding misinformation).[13] The researchers found that although all the study participants were receptive to pseudoscience to some degree, those who reported *greater* trust in science were more likely to believe and disseminate misinformation that contained scientific references than they were misinformation that didn't. If the false facts looked science-ish, they could fool people who had greater overall faith in science. Interestingly, when the researchers reminded participants of the importance of critically evaluating science, it reduced their belief in false claims—whereas being reminded of the value of trusting science did not.

In wellness culture, rife with pseudoscience, simply "trusting science" can be as risky as reflexively dismissing it. Of course few of us have the time or capacity to do a deep dive into the science behind every wellness claim—we can't be experts in everything—so how can you quickly separate solid evidence from pseudoscience, misinterpretations, and other misinformation? Here are a few key strategies for critically evaluating scientific research (and reports about it).

First, see if you can find out any information about the study design. Look for double-blind, randomized controlled trials, or RCTs. Those are the gold standard of evidence when it comes to interventions that claim to promote health and wellness, because double-blind RCTs can tease out what's actually due to the intervention versus what's due to the placebo/nocebo effect, other confounding factors, or simply chance. Our human beliefs and desires, as well as our susceptibility to influence from others, too often cloud our judgment about wellness treatments, making anecdotal evidence an unreliable indicator of whether a given intervention will work for us—or for our patients/clients/ research subjects. (Healthcare providers and even scientists themselves are susceptible to these forms of bias.) We need studies that can effectively control for all that bias, and double-blind RCTs fit the bill.

Yet one challenge with study design—especially in studies that focus on "lifestyle changes" like diet and exercise—is that in some cases it's impossible to conduct double-blind research. That is, sometimes the researchers and/or the participants know what kind of intervention each group is getting, because you can't easily keep people from knowing which foods they're eating or what kind of physical activity they're doing. And studies that are *not* double-blind are vulnerable to placebo effects— beliefs about a diet or exercise plan can favorably influence outcomes.

What's more, RCTs are expensive and time-consuming to conduct, so there aren't a lot of them in the wellness space. Instead, most studies in this area are observational or epidemiological, which means that they can show *correlations* between certain behaviors (such as eating a particular food or taking a particular supplement) and health outcomes, but they can't show *causation*. Unfortunately, even reputable media and health websites often confuse correlation and causation, reporting on epidemiological studies using headlines like "Dark Chocolate Prevents Heart Disease" (WebMD)[14] and "That Morning Cup of Coffee May Extend Your Life" (*U.S. News & World Report*).[15] In many cases, these kinds of correlations can ultimately be explained by social determinants of health and other confounding variables that have nothing to do with the food, supplement, or physical activity in question. (For example, what socioeconomic group is likely to eat dark chocolate regularly? Might they have lower levels of heart disease for other reasons?) But most existing observational studies haven't collected sufficient information on income, race, and other social and behavioral factors that might explain these kinds of associations. So I'd advise taking results from epidemiological studies with a grain of salt.

Moreover, observational studies generally are based on self-reported data, including food-frequency questionnaires (FFQs), which are notoriously unreliable. People often over- or underestimate their consumption of particular foods on questionnaires in an effort to "look good" to researchers, or simply don't accurately remember what they ate months, years, or even decades ago. One study asked women between the ages of 34 and 51 to recall how often they'd consumed different types of dairy in *high school*, and attempted to link that to the women's reports of teenage acne.[16] Most people have a hard time correctly recalling what they ate last week, let alone twenty to thirty years ago.

Not only are self-reports questionable, but FFQs can also produce spurious correlations. For a 2016 investigative report, the data-journalism site *FiveThirtyEight* hired the maker of a respected FFQ to administer its six-month questionnaire to three of the website's writers and a group of reader volunteers. The FFQ company also surveyed participants on various other aspects of their lifestyle, and then *FiveThirtyEight* ran statistical regressions that produced utterly laughable links, including correlations between eating egg rolls and owning a dog, eating table salt and having a positive relationship with your Internet service provider, and eating cabbage and having an innie belly button.[17]

Finally, epidemiological studies rely heavily on measures of relative risk, which can be misleading. Absolute risk describes the overall likelihood of something happening (for example, the risk of developing a certain disease), while relative risk describes the risk of something happening in one group of people versus another. Relative risk statements go something like this: "people who eat flurfengurfens"—an imaginary food I made up—"every day have a 50 percent increased risk of developing colon cancer compared to those who eat flurfengurfens once a week." Relative risk numbers can sound like a lot, and unfortunately people tend to misread statistics like the above as "50 percent of people who eat flurfengurfens will develop colon cancer," which is definitely *not* the case—in fact, the difference in absolute risk between the two groups is remarkably small. For example, the absolute risk of a woman under the age of 50 developing colon and rectal cancer is only four-tenths of a percent (four in one thousand).[18] That would mean that for women under 50 who eat a lot of flurfengurfens, the absolute risk increases to six tenths of a percent (six in one thousand). That change isn't likely to make any meaningful difference in someone's life, even though technically it is a 50 percent increased risk. But bending over backwards to try to avoid that tiny increase in absolute risk can come at a steep cost to one's mental health—and sometimes physical health, too, as is often the case when people go on a diet in an effort to avoid risks and develop disordered eating as a result.

That covers the issues with many genuine scientific studies and the mainstream reporting about them, but what about nontraditional sources? In general, it's helpful to take those, too, with a grain (or perhaps in some cases a spoonful) of salt. If a source is using scientific-sounding terms you've never heard, cross-check them with reputable sources, as discussed. If you don't see those terms in high-impact scientific journals, news reports, or mainstream health websites, you might be in the presence of pseudoscience. And if a source is trying to tell you that they and only they have access to some truth that science hasn't caught up to yet—like the Medical Mediums of the world—it's probably best to steer clear.

*Unplug and Log Off*

Social connection is essential for well-being, but so is solitude. We need time to ourselves, without input from others, to process and make sense of our thoughts, our feelings, our lives. Introverts and extroverts may differ in terms of the *quantity* of alone time we require, but no one functions at their best without quality time on their own. Solitude, unlike isolation, is a necessary counterbalance to connection. And in our hyper-connected world, where every moment of potential downtime is increasingly occupied by input from our digital devices, solitude has become a scarce resource.

In his 2019 book *Digital Minimalism,* computer scientist and author Cal Newport contends that we're in the midst of a solitude shortage brought about by the rise of Internet-enabled smartphones and the hyper-connectedness that goes along with them. He defines *solitude deprivation* as "a state in which you spend close to zero time alone with your own thoughts and free from input from other minds." This deprivation, he argues, reduces our ability to solve problems, to regulate our emotions, and even to strengthen our relationships, because time apart is necessary for creating strong bonds. "If you suffer from chronic solitude deprivation," he writes, "therefore the quality of your life degrades."[19]

In other words, being online all the time can reduce your well-being.

I've talked a lot about technology in this book because it's such a major factor in the spread of harmful wellness-culture ideals and wellness misinformation. And unplugging from technology to the extent that we're able to is helpful in part because it can help stop the spread of such mis- and disinformation. If enough of us take ourselves out of the digital milieu, viral falsehoods won't be able to infect us. And at the societal level, that virus will have fewer hosts and won't be able to travel as far.

Clearly there's a limit to how effective this practice can be in creating large-scale social change, since individual users of technology are up against powerful platforms designed to keep us addicted (or "engaged") for profit, as we've discussed—which is why first and foremost we need structural, policy-level changes to make the Internet a safer place. But in the meantime, if we can reduce our dependence on technology enough to reclaim some measure of solitude and thereby strengthen our emotion-regulation skills, we might make ourselves a little less vulnerable to online mis- and disinformation (about wellness or anything else) whenever we do come across it. Having the ability to stop, breathe, and reflect before reflexively jumping into outrage and hitting "share" can help keep us—and those around us—from being exposed to harmful content.

When thinking about reducing social media and Internet use (or taking a break from digital devices altogether), one thing that often comes up for people is a fear of missing out on content that could help us learn and grow. "Doing your research" has become synonymous with online practices like googling and "following" social media content creators—to the extent that it's difficult to imagine other ways of learning if you're not formally in school. But in fact there's a whole world of possibilities for developing knowledge beyond just scrolling. Natalia Mehlman Petrzela, the wellness-culture historian, points out that having conversations with actual people in your life—those you respect and trust, and whose opinions you value, even if you don't always agree with them—is an important way to come to new understandings. These conversations can help you "refine your thinking and your sense of self and your perspective," she says. "I think of those human connections as a way to stay grounded and keep a healthy skepticism that doesn't devolve into conspiracism, and we should work hard to cultivate those."

Not having—or losing track of—those real-world relationships can leave you vulnerable to the extremism that proliferates online. Heather Simpson, the former anti-vax influencer we met in Chapter 5, knows that all too well. "I think when I was so in the online world, I forgot that normal people existed," she says. Essentially her whole social milieu became the anti-vax movement, with relationships that existed almost entirely online. Hundreds of people would "like" her anti-vax status updates. It wasn't until she got out that she realized how comparatively tiny that world really is. "Even though it felt like it was a ton of people, it's actually a really small amount of people, and most of the world is pro-vax," she says.

Unfortunately, the COVID years pushed many people to conduct their social lives primarily online, out of necessity. That created a situation where many of us experienced both profound isolation and solitude deprivation — being at once cut off from real-world human connection and digitally hyper-connected, making it hard to find space to hear ourselves think. In some ways, online connections were a lifeline for many people in a time of isolation; being able to stay in touch with people far away became more important than ever, especially for those who live alone. And yet the type of discourse this hyper-online-ness created was harmful to many people's well-being. Instead of in-depth discussions with people you trusted, it was often surface-level communications and comment flame wars with strangers. When algorithms amplify outrage and hot takes, genuine human connections are thwarted.

In the past few years, I've personally taken a big step back from social media, though I still spend a fair amount of time online reading the news and researching for my writing. I've tried to go back to treating the Internet like a library — a place to find quality information and occasionally email people — as I did decades ago, before social media. I've cultivated more solitude and real-world connections. I've become less interested in people's hot takes on the news — or in what they're saying about me—than I am in protecting my mental and emotional well-being. And I've felt a major positive shift as a result.

I know that unplugging entirely from social platforms may not be desirable or even possible for everyone, and I recognize that in many ways it's a privilege to be able to choose to log off. But to the extent you're able to, you might consider ways to reduce your use of these technologies—particularly the wellness-culture corners of social media—and see if it helps you feel more grounded, stable, and present in other areas of your life. It doesn't have to be an all-or-nothing proposition, and you can experiment with ways to reduce your time on the platforms, starting as small as you want.

Regardless of whether you take a full-on break from social media, know that targeted ads for diets and other wellness-culture products will likely continue to follow you around the Internet until you start using ad-blocking software, which I'd recommend doing if you're not already. Pair that with a privacy-focused search engine such as DuckDuckGo, log off from any social media accounts you're not actively using, and clear your browser history and cache often, and you'll likely start seeing far fewer ads. If you do continue to see them, most ad servers allow you to flag or report them as inappropriate, which theoretically should tell the server to show you fewer ads like that in the future. And of course it helps to unfollow and unsubscribe from any wellness-culture influencers who are serving up misinformation. In fact, I'd consider trying not to take *any* health or wellness advice from social media if you can help it, because the algorithms can push even thoughtful, credentialed healthcare providers to write and speak in less-nuanced ways than they otherwise would.

*Heal from Wellness Culture*

If you've fallen into the wellness trap and been harmed by it, finding support for your healing is key. As Simpson explains, having at least one supportive friend was instrumental in helping her come out of the fog of mis- and disinformation. This was a close friend who continued to have in-depth conversations with her even while she was at her most entrenched in the anti-vax movement. "She was very gentle, but she was very truthful, and she never got fed up with me for two years," Simpson says. Instead of debating Simpson or coming at her with an accusatory tone, the way so many people online did, her friend was empathetic and treated her like a human being. That approach was incredibly powerful. "I was able to actually open up and listen to what she was saying," Simpson says. It helped her feel safe enough to eventually reconsider her views, though that process took time.

What if you haven't gotten drawn into the anti-vaccine world as Simpson did, but instead got labeled with a dubious diagnosis and prescribed spurious cures, like the people we met in Chapter 6? You might consider finding new providers if you're ready, as well as addressing the harm caused by previous treatments, including their effect on your mental well-being. I know that's a lot easier said than done in a healthcare system that may already have failed you in many ways, and allowing yourself to grieve for everything you've been through is an important first step.

It also can be helpful to remember that if you've been let down by alternative-, integrative-, and functional-medicine providers, there's no shame in giving conventional medicine another try. Despite the many flaws in the system, there are medical professionals out there who are compassionate and kind, who rely on the best available scientific evidence and won't push misinformation. Contrary to what wellness conspiracy theories would have you believe, all doctors aren't uncaring monsters who are just in it for the money. Most of them genuinely do want to help and are happy to share what they know, not keep secrets for profit. Granted, truly great medical providers may not always be easy to find—or to access, depending on your economic situation and your insurance coverage—and that's frustrating and unjust. Sometimes finding a good fit is a game of trial and error, which can be time-consuming and emotionally draining, as I know from experience. But in many cases you do have a choice, and you certainly don't have to stick with an alternative-medicine provider whose prescriptions don't seem to be effective, even if they try to assure you that feeling worse means their protocol is working.

If pursuing wellness-culture "cures" has led you down a path of disordered eating, overexercise, and/or poor body image, there is help available. Again, because the American healthcare system in particular is so problematic, such specialized help may not always be accessible, which is another thing that needs to be addressed at the systemic and policy level. But under American healthcare parity laws, all insurance policies are at least required to cover mental-health care at the same level they do for physical-health care—meaning that for mental and emotional conditions like disordered eating, psychotherapy and sessions with a registered dietitian should be covered. If you're struggling and you have access to these services, I highly recommend using them to help you heal. (As a starting point, I have a list of providers who treat disordered eating at christyharrison.com/providers.)

Learning to practice self-compassion while experiencing discomfort is also key. Meditation teacher and author Sebene Selassie, who has survived multiple bouts of cancer, has written about "meeting each moment of pain as an opportunity for well-being."[20] As she wrote in 2021, one side effect of her latest cancer treatment was intense pain in her joints, nerves, and muscles. Very quickly, she started to imagine that the pain was going to be progressive and permanent, and to see it as a failure on her part. She believed it was her fault for not doing enough wellness-culture practices, or not doing them in the "right" way, or doing too much of certain things at the expense of others. Although pain in and of itself is merely a signal that something in the body needs attention, "I packed the pain with judgment and reactivity, with doubt and dismay," she wrote. "I was letting my lack of wellness decrease my well-being." Eventually, she began to practice noticing the pain without judgment, offering herself compassion for what she was going through, and finding small ways to help herself feel better, without the sense of fault or self-blame. Although wellness culture's idea of wellness (total physical and mental optimization) was out of reach for her, as it is for so many of us, she still was able to access some measure of well-being.

### Social Connection, Boundaries, and Purpose

In advocating reducing your dependence on social media, I'm by no means recommending total social disconnection (as much as it may feel that way, because social media has come to stand in for so much connection, particularly during the pandemic). Just as solitude is essential for well-being, so is social connectedness—and there are ways to get it without social media. Many studies, including several reviews and meta-analyses over the past decade or so, have found that positive social relationships, frequent social contact, and strong family ties are protective for well-being, and for longevity.[21]

Lack of social connection is a risk factor for poor mental and physical health. Other, related risk factors include loneliness, divorce, and widowhood. Research controlling for initial health status (and of course age and other factors) shows that people who are more socially connected are at significantly lower risk of disease, mental-health problems, and death, and that those who are less socially connected are at significantly higher risk (though there aren't any RCTs to prove that greater social connection *causes* better well-being, or that lack of connection *causes* worse outcomes).

Interestingly, lacking in social connectedness has been shown to be an equal or greater risk factor for mortality than "obesity," which is a reminder that anti-fat bias and the social isolation it creates is a major missing factor in the scientific research on weight and health. How much of the risk supposedly attributable to high BMI is actually the result of loneliness and disconnection caused by weight stigma? And of course social isolation was only exacerbated by the pandemic, for people across the weight spectrum.

But it's not enough just to have social connection; we need *quality* social connection. When our close relationships are full of conflict and strife, it can detract from overall well-being. Although some research has found that online social connection, such as that fostered by social media, is associated with beneficial outcomes, we've seen how online connectedness can go terribly wrong amid wellness culture and a social media environment that thrives on outrage and division. Social connection that becomes a source of misinformation and conspiracy theories undoubtedly has a net-negative impact on well-being.

For some of us, cultivating supportive relationships might entail getting some help in therapy to overcome harmful patterns of relating (though again, there are many barriers to accessing therapy that need to be addressed at the systemic level). Another important aspect of building strong relationships is setting necessary boundaries—including, perhaps, conveying to the wellness-culture adherents in your life that you love and support them but that you're on a different path. If friends and family members can't stop talking about their latest "wellness plan," "candida cleanse," or "autoimmune protocol," you might share with them that those types of things have been harmful to you in the past, and that in order to protect your own healing you'd rather not hear about them.

Although we've talked a lot in this book about the lack of scientific evidence to support many wellness-culture "cures," getting into the science may not land well with people who are currently invested in these approaches. Instead, I've often found it helpful to stay focused on your own story and your own needs, since the people who care about you typically will respect those (and generally want to do their best to understand and support you).

It is also important to recognize why people get caught up in wellness culture, and to have empathy for those who embrace it. For many of us, it starts with feeling disappointed, unheard, or excluded by the Western medical system. Most people can probably remember at least one time, if not many, when they felt this way about conventional medicine. As we've discussed, wellness culture is expert at swooping in and offering "solutions" (sometimes in good faith, sometimes not) when people are in a vulnerable state. These supposed cures often don't work and may actively cause harm, but once you've gotten caught in the wellness trap it can be hard to untangle yourself.

Wellness culture can do a great job of giving people a sense of purpose. Having an identity as a "wellness warrior" bravely fighting illness and disease with food and supplements alone — and perhaps also as a wellness *purveyor*, selling products advertised as lifesaving — can help people make meaning out of their struggles. That's hugely appealing, and it's no wonder people are drawn in by it. Having a sense of meaning and purpose is a major component of well-being, and it's completely understandable why we'd seek that out.

In fact, in cultivating a sense of purpose outside of wellness culture, we might help make ourselves a little less vulnerable to falling into its traps.

Over the past decade or two, research has shown the benefits of finding purpose in life. "The extent to which individuals see their lives as having meaning, a sense of direction, and goals to live for," write the authors of one study, "...is often viewed as central to well-being and fulfillment."[22] For example, a 2022 study in a large, nationally representative sample of nearly thirteen thousand U.S. adults over the age of fifty found that over a four-year follow-up period, the participants with the highest (versus lowest) sense of purpose had better psychological and social outcomes, including significantly higher levels of optimism, lower levels of loneliness, and a 43 percent reduced risk of depression and a 16 percent reduced risk of cognitive impairment.[23] They also had better physical health outcomes, notably including a 46 percent reduced risk of mortality, fewer chronic conditions, and higher self-rated health. This was correlational data, so again, we can't say that purpose in life *caused* better well-being. But the researchers did control for an impressive variety of variables—among them race/ethnicity, annual household income, total wealth, level of education, employment status, health insurance, prior experiences of childhood abuse, preexisting chronic disease, and life purpose prior to the study period—making it more likely that the results can't entirely be explained by these other factors.

As for *how* to build purpose in life, that's an open question. A few RCTs have explored whether interventions such as volunteering and specific types of group therapy can help to increase one's sense of purpose, but the results have been mixed and studies have been small, with some showing that such interventions have no effect.[24] Perhaps that's because a sense of purpose and meaning is unique to each individual and can't be imposed from the outside. Instead, purpose is something that has to be discovered, through some combination of life experience and solitary reflection. And your sense of purpose is likely to change and evolve through the years.

You may once have felt, as I did, that your primary purpose in life was to pursue self-optimization through various avenues offered by wellness culture—only to realize later that that pursuit was in fact standing in the way of authentic meaning and purpose. Of course, part of my search for physical improvement was driven by an understandable desire to heal from my chronic illnesses and stop the suffering they were causing. But there were other, more noxious layers to it as well. At some level I thought I needed to be free from symptoms and functioning "optimally" in order to be worthy. I thought that not fitting wellness culture's perfectionistic ideal of health—wrapped up as it is in Eurocentric standards of beauty and thinness—made me less desirable, less feminine, and therefore less deserving of love and intimacy. I thought my struggles with chronic illness meant that I wouldn't be able to succeed as a nutrition journalist or, later, as a dietitian—because if I was really good at those jobs, I would have figured out how to "heal myself with food." I knew I wasn't alone in dealing with chronic conditions—far from it—and yet deep down I felt that I needed to completely erase them in order to fulfill the dreams I had for my life. And so in some ways, the quest for wellness started to stand in for those dreams. It went from being the path to achieving my purpose, to feeling like the purpose itself. Like so many people who get caught in the rigid confines of wellness culture, my life became organized around the quest for an unattainable ideal.

In my view, that's not what it means to be "well"; in fact, quite the opposite. Instead of inflexible standards, we need the freedom to discover our purpose in life, and to experience all the other elements that make up well-being. But that's not available to everyone in our current discriminatory, economically unequal, hypercompetitive, optimization-driven society. Wellness culture is not the path to achieving meaning, joy, relatedness; it's just one of many obstacles standing in the way. Ultimately, we need change at the systemic and cultural levels to create the conditions for *true* well-being—a state not of striving for "perfect" physical and mental health, but rather one of social support, economic security, just and equitable treatment, purpose, and satisfaction in life. Because that's what everyone deserves.

# Acknowledgments

I am profoundly grateful to Marisa Vigilante, my editor at Little, Brown Spark, for her incisive yet gentle guidance and her clear-eyed vision of what this book could become. Thanks to Spark publisher Tracy Behar for believing in this project; to Maria Espinosa, David Coen, and Linda Arends for elevating it from a manuscript to a finished book; to Lucy Kim for giving it an eye-catching cover; and to Jessica Chun, Juliana Horbachevsky, Fanta Diallo, and Bruce Nichols for helping it find its audience.

My agent, Brettne Bloom, made this book possible and provided invaluable feedback along the way. Kelly Diels was instrumental in helping outline the proposal.

I'm deeply indebted to Janet Byrne for her expert fact checking and perceptive edits, which made this book immeasurably better. I never would have been able to wrangle all the research that went into this project without the help of Jeanette Miller, Katie Dalebout, Alex Van Buren, Cynthia Vazquez, and Woo-Jin Jung.

Jenée Desmond-Harris, Jonathan Vatner, Alex Garinger, and Maria Grasso offered thoughtful comments on early drafts, helping to add layers of compassion and nuance to the narrative. My writer-moms group—Sarah, Lacy, Lesley, Apryl, and Helen—provided brilliant insights and moral support as the book neared completion.

My sincerest gratitude to everyone I interviewed for this book, including those whose stories I wasn't able to include.

Your input helped inform my thinking on wellness culture, and I'm honored that you shared your experiences with me, even when some of them were no doubt challenging to re-live.

Julianne Wotasik, Vincci Tsui, Mike Lalonde, Mycroft Holmes, Lauren Giammarella, and Abigail Haynes helped keep my business running smoothly so that I could focus on writing. Marcia and Abby C. helped me carve out time for revisions in those hazy postpartum months.

Mom, Dad, Ma, Pops, Midge, Burt, Pete, and Colin, your love and support means the world to me. To my husband, my best friend and first reader, thank you for taking care of me and our family in countless ways, large and small. I couldn't have written this, or much of anything, without you. And to my daughter, you inspire me every day to imagine a better world and work to bring it into being. I can't wait to see who you become.

# Notes

Interviewees quoted in this book include (in alphabetical order): Maxine Ali, Susanna Barkataki, Roberta Blevins, Renée DiResta, Karen Douglas, Anita Emly, Jody Esselstyn, William Keep, Chrissy King, Erin Lemley, Máire O Sullivan, Asher Pandjiris, Natalia Mehlman Petrzela, El Poché, Carolyn Roberts, Dawn Serra, Heather Simpson, Kate Spies, Erin Todd, and Julian Walker, as well as several sources in Chapter 6 who asked to use pseudonyms or first names only. All quotes from these sources not otherwise attributed are from my conversations with them.

### *Introduction*
1. Sun Jae Jung et al., "Posttraumatic Stress Disorder and Incidence of Thyroid Dysfunction in Women.," *Psychological Medicine* 49, no. 15 (2019): 2551–60, https://doi.org/10.1017/S0033291718003495.
2. Qin Xiang Ng et al., "Systematic Review with Meta-Analysis: The Association between Post-Traumatic Stress Disorder and Irritable Bowel Syndrome.," *Journal of Gastroenterology and Hepatology* 34, no. 1 (January 2019): 68–73, https://doi.org/10.1111/jgh.14446.
3. Risa B Weisberg et al., "Nonpsychiatric Illness among Primary Care Patients with Trauma Histories and Posttraumatic Stress Disorder.," *Psychiatric Services (Washington, D.C.)* 53, no. 7 (July 2002): 848–54, https://doi.org/10.1176/appi.ps.53.7.848.
4. National Center for Chronic Disease, "Chronic Diseases in America | CDC," CDC.gov, 2021, https://www.cdc.gov/chronicdisease/resources/infographic/chronic-diseases.htm.
5. Ronald L Simons et al., "Racial Discrimination, Inflammation, and Chronic Illness Among African American Women at Midlife: Support for the Weathering Perspective.," *Journal of Racial and Ethnic Health Disparities*, June 3, 2020, https://doi.org/10.1007/s40615-020-00786-8.

6. Kevin Miscella and Mechelle R Sanders, "Racial and Ethnic Disparities in the Quality of Health Care.," *Annual Review of Public Health* 37 (2016): 375–94, https://doi.org/10.1146/annurev-publhealth-032315-021439.

7. Akilah Johnson and Dan Keating, "Whites Now More Likely to Die from Covid than Blacks: Why the Pandemic Shifted," *The Washington Post*, October 19, 2022, https://www.washingtonpost.com/health/2022/10/19/covid-deaths-us-race/.

8. Ahmad Chandiramani, "Racial, Ethnic, and Socioeconomic Disparities in Confirmed COVID-19 Cases and Deaths in the United States: A County-Level Analysis as of November 2020," *Ethnicity & Health* 26, no. 1 (January 2, 2021): 22–35, https://doi.org/10.1080/13557858.2020.1853067.

9. Global Wellness Institute, "What Is Wellness?," accessed April 1, 2021, https://globalwellnessinstitute.org/what-is-wellness/.

10. Rachel Syme, "Puzzling Through Our Eternal Quest for Wellness," *The New Yorker*, March 22, 2021, https://www.newyorker.com/magazine/2021/03/29/puzzling-through-our-eternal-quest-for-wellness.

11. Kate Berlant and Jacqueline Novak, "Introducing: POOG," *POOG Podcast*, November 9, 2020, https://www.iheart.com/podcast/1119-poog-with-kate-berlant-an-73595748/episode/introducing-poog-73595764/.

12. Global Wellness Institute, "2022 The Global Wellness Economy: Country Rankings," 2022, https://globalwellnessinstitute.org/industry-research/2022-global-wellness-economy-country-rankings/

13. Shaun Callaghan et al., "The Future of the $1.5 Trillion Wellness Market," April 8, 2021, https://www.mckinsey.com/industries/consumer-packaged-goods/our-insights/feeling-good-the-future-of-the-1-5-trillion-wellness-market.

14. Global Wellness Institute, "Defining the Mental Wellness Economy 2020," November 2020, https://globalwellnessinstitute.org/defining-the-mental-wellness-economy-2020/.

15. Jackie Chequeen, "The Effects of COVID-19 on the Wellness Industry," *CO by U.S. Chamber of Commerce*, August 11, 2020, https://www.uschamber.com/co/good-company/launch-pad/pandemic-is-changing-wellness-industry.

16. Christy Harrison, *Anti-Diet: Reclaim Your Time, Money, Well-Being, and Happiness Through Intuitive Eating* (New York: Little, Brown Spark, 2019).

17. Michaela C Pascoe, David R Thompson, and Chantal F Ski, "Yoga, Mindfulness-Based Stress Reduction and Stress-Related Physiological Measures: A Meta-Analysis.," *Psychoneuroendocrinology* 86 (December 2017): 152–68, https://doi.org/10.1016/j.psyneuen.2017.08.008; Autumn M Gallegos et al., "Meditation and Yoga for Posttraumatic Stress Disorder: A Meta-Analytic Review of Randomized Controlled Trials.," *Clinical Psychology Review* 58 (December 2017): 115–24, https://doi.org/10.1016/j.cpr.2017.10.004.

18. Madhav Goyal et al., "Meditation Programs for Psychological Stress and Well-Being: A Systematic Review and Meta-Analysis.," *JAMA Internal*

*Medicine* 174, no. 3 (March 2014): 357–68, https://doi.org/10.1001/jama
internmed.2013.13018.

### Chapter 1: Wellness and Diet Culture

1. Halbert L. Dunn, "What High-Level Wellness Means," *Canadian Journal of Public Health* 50, no. 11 (1959): 447–57, https://www.jstor.org/stable /41981469?seq=1.
2. Halbert L. Dunn, "High-Level Wellness for Man and Society.," *American Journal of Public Health and the Nation's Health* 49, no. 6 (June 1959): 786– 92, https://doi.org/10.2105/ajph.49.6.786.
3. Ben Zimmer, "On Language: Wellness," *The New York Times*, April 16, 2010, https://www.nytimes.com/2010/04/18/magazine/18FOB-onlangu age-t.html.
4. Rose Wunrow, "The Psychological Massacre: Jim Jones and Peoples Temple: An Investigation," Department of Religious Studies at San Diego State University, https://jonestown.sdsu.edu/?page_id=29478; Dave Mitchell, Cathy Mitchell, and Richard Ofshe, *The Light of Synanon: How a Country Weekly Exposed a Corporate Cult—and Won the Pulitzer Prize* (New York: Seaview Books, 1980); Jeffrey Klein, "Reading Helen Palmer," *Mother Jones*, April 1979, 58–63, https://books.google.com/books?id=pOYDAA AAMBAJ&pg=PA58&lpg=PA58&dq=church+of+divine+man+motherjo nes&source=bl&ots=26bROMltjR&sig=2rL2MoV41iBkARzEPsoP6l6G7x A&hl=en&sa=X&ved=0ahUKEwiw38KQ9ZrVAhXjxFQKHemICGgQ6A EILTAB#v=onepage&q=church%20of%20divine%20man%20 motherjones&f=false.
5. "Wellness Resource Center with Dan Rather on *60 Minutes*," November 1979, https://www.youtube.com/watch?v=LAorj2U7PR4.
6. Jonathan Kauffman, *Hippie Food: How Back-to-the-Landers, Longhairs, and Revolutionaries Changed the Way We Eat* (New York: William Morrow, 2018).
7. The term "orthorexia nervosa" was introduced in 1996 by the American doctor Steven Bratman, who published a book covering the subject four years later: Steven Bratman with David Knight, *Health Food Junkies: Overcoming the Obsession with Healthful Eating* (New York: Broadway Books, 2000), 5–92.
8. Donald B. Ardell, *High Level Wellness: An Alternative to Doctors, Drugs, and Disease* (Emmaus, PA: Rodale Press, 1977), 118, 50.
9. Sabrina Strings, *Fearing the Black Body: The Racial Origins of Fat Phobia*, 1st ed. (New York: New York University Press, 2019), https://nyupress.org /books/9781479886753/.
10. Michael Greger with Gene Stone, *How Not to Die: Discover the Food Scientifically Proven to Prevent and Reverse Disease* (New York: Flatiron Books, 2015).
11. Tula Karras, "Disordered Eating: The Disorder next Door," *SELF*, April 20, 2008, https://www.self.com/story/eating-disorder-risk.
12. See E. W. Diemer et al., "Beyond the Binary: Differences in Eating Disorder Prevalence by Gender Identity in a Transgender Sample," *Transgender Health* 3, no. 1, 17–23.

13. Jason M. Nagata et al., "Predictors of Muscularity-oriented Disordered Eating Behaviors in U.S. Young Adults: A Prospective Cohort Study," *International Journal of Eating Disorders* 52, no. 12 (December 20, 2019): 1380–88, https://doi.org/10.1002/eat.23094.

14. Marie Galmiche et al., "Prevalence of Eating Disorders over the 2000–2018 Period: A Systematic Literature Review," *The American Journal of Clinical Nutrition* 109, no. 5 (May 1, 2019): 1402–13, https://doi.org/10.1093/ajcn/nqy342.

15. Gholamreza Khaksar, Kitipong Assatarakul, and Supaart Sirikantaramas, "Effect of Cold-Pressed and Normal Centrifugal Juicing on Quality Attributes of Fresh Juices: Do Cold-Pressed Juices Harbor a Superior Nutritional Quality and Antioxidant Capacity?," *Heliyon* 5, no. 6 (June 2019): e01917, https://doi.org/10.1016/j.heliyon.2019.e01917.

16. Gildeilza Gomes Silva et al., "Processing Methods with Heat Increases Bioactive Phenolic Compounds and Antioxidant Activity in Grape Juices.," *Journal of Food Biochemistry* 43, no. 3 (2019): e12732, https://doi.org/10.1111/jfbc.12732.

17. Gabi Conti, "The Science Behind The Celery Juice Trend," *MindBodyGreen*, October 7, 2019, https://www.mindbodygreen.com/articles/science-behind-celery-juice-trend.

18. "Labelling—Food Allergy and Food Intolerance—CCEA," BBC, accessed April 13, 2021, https://www.bbc.co.uk/bitesize/guides/z23yfcw/revision/5.

19. Lauren Williamson, "The Celery Juice Trend Could Be Putting Your Health at Risk," *Australian Women's Health*, April 5, 2019, https://www.womenshealth.com.au/celery-juice-trend-health-risks. And M C A Polderman et al., "A Double-Blind Placebo-Controlled Trial of UVA-1 in the Treatment of Dyshidrotic Eczema.," *Clinical and Experimental Dermatology* 28, no. 6 (November 2003): 584–87, https://doi.org/10.1046/j.1365-2230.2003.01378.x.

20. JS Berg and JL Moore, "A Case of 'Eating Disorder NOS': Aeromedical Implications of DSM-IV Diagnostic Criteria," *Aviation, Space, and Environmental Medicine* 67, no. 2 (1996): 157–60.

21. Molli Mitchell, "Who Is Elise Loehnen and Why Did She Leave Gwyneth Paltrow's Goop?," *Newsweek*, March 25, 2022, https://www.newsweek.com/why-did-elise-leohnen-leave-goop-gwyneth-paltrow-cleanse-instagram-1691759.

22. U.S. Food and Drug Administration, "FDA Investigation into Potential Link between Certain Diets and Canine Dilated Cardiomyopathy," fda.gov, June 27, 2019, https://www.fda.gov/animal-veterinary/outbreaks-and-advisories/fda-investigation-potential-link-between-certain-diets-and-canine-dilated-cardiomyopathy.

23. WSAVA Global Nutrition Committee, "Frequently Asked Questions & Myths," World Small Animal Veterinary Association, 2018, https://wsava.org/wp-content/uploads/2020/01/Frequently-Asked-Questions-and-Myths.pdf.

24. Linda Carroll, "After FDA Warning about Grain-Free Pet Food, What's Safe to Feed Our Pets?," *NBC News*, July 8, 2019, https://www.nbcnews

.com/health/health-news/after-fda-warning-about-grain-free-pet-food
-what-s-n1026881.

25. Whitney Akers, "Annual Gym Membership: Worth It?," *Healthline*, September 24, 2018, https://www.healthline.com/health-news/gym-member ships-can-be-a-trap. And Cory Stieg, "Why Fitness Classes Cost So Much More Than Gym Workouts," *Refinery29*, February 6, 2019, https://www .refinery29.com/en-us/fitness-classes-cost-expensive.

26. Katherine Rosman, "CrossFit Gyms Founder Resigns Amid Black Lives Matter Furor," *The New York Times*, June 9, 2020, https://www.nytimes .com/2020/06/09/style/crossfit-gyms-founder-protests.html.

27. Katie Warren, "SoulCycle's Top Instructors Had Sex with Clients, 'Fat-Shamed' Coworkers, and Used Homophobic and Racist Language, but the Company Treated Them Like Hollywood Stars Anyway, Insiders Say," *Business Insider*, November 17, 2020, https://web.archive.org/web/2021 0213055125/https://www.businessinsider.com/soulcycle-instructors -celebrities-misbehavior-2020-11.

28. Chantal M Koolhaas et al., "Impact of Physical Activity on the Association of Overweight and Obesity with Cardiovascular Disease: The Rotterdam Study.," *European Journal of Preventive Cardiology* 24, no. 9 (2017): 934–41, https://doi.org/10.1177/2047487317693952.

29. Vaughn W. Barry et al., "Fitness vs. Fatness on All-Cause Mortality: A Meta-Analysis," *Progress in Cardiovascular Diseases* 56, no. 4 (January 1, 2014): 382–90, https://doi.org/10.1016/J.PCAD.2013.09.002.

30. Glenn A. Gaesser and Siddhartha S. Angadi, "Obesity Treatment: Weight Loss versus Increasing Fitness and Physical Activity for Reducing Health Risks," *IScience* 24, no. 10 (October 22, 2021): 102995, https://doi.org /10.1016/j.isci.2021.102995.

31. Cory Stieg, "Twitter CEO Jack Dorsey: 'I Eat Seven Meals Every Week, Just Dinner,'" CNBC, January 15, 2020, https://www.cnbc.com/2020/01/15 /twitter-ceo-jack-dorsey-eats-seven-meals-every-week-only-dinner.html.

32. Monica Hesse, "The Key to Glorifying a Questionable Diet? Be a Tech Bro and Call It 'Biohacking.,'" *The Washington Post*, April 11, 2019, https://www.washingtonpost.com/lifestyle/style/the-key-to-glorify ing-a-questionable-diet-be-a-tech-bro-and-call-it-biohacking/2019/04 /11/12368e2c-5ba2-11e9-842d-7d3ed7eb3957_story.html.

33. Olivia Solon, "The Silicon Valley Execs Who Don't Eat for Days: 'It's Not Dieting, It's Biohacking,'" *The Guardian*, September 4, 2017, https:// www.theguardian.com/lifeandstyle/2017/sep/04/silicon-valley-ceo-fast ing-trend-diet-is-it-safe.

34. Julia Malacoff, "Everything You Need to Know About Biohacking Your Body," *Shape*, April 9, 2018, https://www.shape.com/healthy-eating/diet -tips/what-is-biohacking-nutrition-science.

35. "Playing God in Your Basement," *The Washington Post*, January 31, 1988, https://www.washingtonpost.com/archive/opinions/1988/01/31 /playing-god-in-your-basement/618f174d-fc11-47b3-a8db-fae1b8340c67 /?noredirect=on&utm_term=.7c36c72844ba.

36. Deying Liu et al., "Calorie Restriction with or without Time-Restricted Eating in Weight Loss," *New England Journal of Medicine* 386, no. 16 (April 21, 2022): 1495–1504, https://doi.org/10.1056/NEJMoa2114833. And Dylan A. Lowe et al., "Effects of Time-Restricted Eating on Weight Loss and Other Metabolic Parameters in Women and Men With Overweight and Obesity," *JAMA Internal Medicine* 180, no. 11 (November 1, 2020): 1491, https://doi.org/10.1001/jamainternmed.2020.4153.

37. Christina Farr, "Intermittent Fasting Doesn't Help Weight Loss: UCSF Study," *CNBC*, September 28, 2020, https://www.cnbc.com/2020/09/28/intermittent-fasting-doesnt-help-weight-loss-ucsf-study.html.

38. Markham Heid, "You Asked: What Is My Poo Telling Me?" *Time*, December 10, 2014, https://time.com/3625206/poop-health/.

39. John M Kelso, "Unproven Diagnostic Tests for Adverse Reactions to Foods.," *The Journal of Allergy and Clinical Immunology. In Practice* 6, no. 2 (March 1, 2018): 362–65, https://doi.org/10.1016/j.jaip.2017.08.021.

40. Bruce A Gingras and Jack A Maggiore, "Performance of a New Molecular Assay for the Detection of Gastrointestinal Pathogens.," *Access Microbiology* 2, no. 10 (2020): acmi000160, https://doi.org/10.1099/acmi.0.000160.

41. Monica Heisey, "This Man Thinks He Never Has to Eat Again," *Vice*, March 13, 2013, https://www.vice.com/en/article/yv59ab/rob-rhinehart-no-longer-requires-food.

### Chapter 2: Clean and Natural

1. Bobbi Brown with Sara Bliss, *Beauty from the Inside Out* (San Francisco: Chronicle Books, 2017).

2. Britta de Pessemier et al., "Gut-Skin Axis: Current Knowledge of the Interrelationship between Microbial Dysbiosis and Skin Conditions.," *Microorganisms* 9, no. 2 (February 11, 2021), https://doi.org/10.3390/microorganisms9020353.

3. Scarlett Dixon, "The Inside-Out Guide to Getting Your Skin to Glow," Healthline, April 16, 2019, https://www.healthline.com/health/guide-how-to-make-skin-glow.

4. Emily Kirkpatrick, "Gwyneth Paltrow Won't Do Botox Again, But She Will Endorse This Anti-Wrinkle Injectable," *Vanity Fair*, September 17, 2020, https://www.vanityfair.com/style/2020/09/gwyneth-paltrow-injectable-anti-wrinkle-beauty-goop.

5. "Goop Lab Vampire Facial with Gwyneth Paltrow," February 10, 2020, https://www.youtube.com/watch?v=uYXlEzNaY0A; Bee Shapiro, "Gwyneth Paltrow Shares Beauty Advice, Even Though Her Daughter Is the Expert," *New York Times*, April 4, 2016, https://www.nytimes.com/2016/04/07/fashion/gwyneth-paltrow-juice-beauty-goop.html?smid=tw-nytimes&smtyp=cur&_r=1.

6. Suzan Obagi, "Why Does Skin Wrinkle with Age? What Is the Best Way to Slow or Prevent This Process?," *Scientific American*, September 26, 2005, https://www.scientificamerican.com/article/why-does-skin-wrinkle-wit/.

7. Rebecca Guenard, "The Allergens in Natural Beauty Products," *The Atlantic*, January 21, 2015, https://www.theatlantic.com/health/archive/2015/01/the-allergens-in-natural-beauty-products/384326/.
8. Molly Fischer, "Will the Millennial Aesthetic Ever End?," *New York Magazine*, March 3, 2020, https://www.thecut.com/2020/03/will-the-millennial-aesthetic-ever-end.html.
9. Elizabeth A. O'Connor et al., *Vitamin, Mineral, and Multivitamin Supplementation for the Primary Prevention of Cardiovascular Disease and Cancer: A Systematic Evidence Review for the U.S. Preventive Services Task Force, Vitamin, Mineral, and Multivitamin Supplementation for the Primary Prevention of Cardiovascular Disease and Cancer: A Systematic Evidence Review for the U.S. Preventive Services Task Force* (Agency for Healthcare Research and Quality (US), 2021), http://www.ncbi.nlm.nih.gov/pubmed/35767665.
10. Roberto Marchioli et al., "Vitamin E Increases the Risk of Developing Heart Failure after Myocardial Infarction: Results from the GISSI-Prevenzione Trial.," *Journal of Cardiovascular Medicine (Hagerstown, Md.)* 7, no. 5 (May 2006): 347–50, https://doi.org/10.2459/01.JCM.0000223257.09062.17.
11. Eric A Klein et al., "Vitamin E and the Risk of Prostate Cancer: The Selenium and Vitamin E Cancer Prevention Trial (SELECT).," *JAMA* 306, no. 14 (October 12, 2011): 1549–56, https://doi.org/10.1001/jama.2011.1437.
12. Marcela Cortés-Jofré et al., "Drugs for Preventing Lung Cancer in Healthy People," *Cochrane Database of Systematic Reviews* 2020, no. 3 (March 4, 2020), https://doi.org/10.1002/14651858.CD002141.pub3.
13. Anahad O'Connor, "Study Warns of Diet Supplement Dangers Kept Quiet by F.D.A.," *The New York Times*, April 7, 2015, https://well.blogs.nytimes.com/2015/04/07/study-warns-of-diet-supplement-dangers-kept-quiet-by-f-d-a/.
14. Pieter A. Cohen et al., "Nine Prohibited Stimulants Found in Sports and Weight Loss Supplements: Deterenol, Phenpromethamine (Vonedrine), Oxilofrine, Octodrine, Beta-Methylphenylethylamine (BMPEA), 1,3-Dimethylamylamine (1,3-DMAA), 1,4-Dimethylamylamine (1,4-DMAA), 1,3-Dimethylbutylamine (1,3-DMBA) and Higenamine," *Clinical Toxicology*, March 23, 2021, 1–7, https://doi.org/10.1080/15563650.2021.1894333.
15. Victor J Navarro et al., "Liver Injury from Herbal and Dietary Supplements.," *Hepatology (Baltimore, Md.)* 65, no. 1 (2017): 363–73, https://doi.org/10.1002/hep.28813.
16. Andrew I. Geller et al., "Emergency Department Visits for Adverse Events Related to Dietary Supplements," *New England Journal of Medicine* 373, no. 16 (October 15, 2015): 1531–40, https://doi.org/10.1056/NEJMsa1504267..
17. Dann Gallucci and Jane Marie, "S2 E4: Take With Caution," *The Dream* podcast, 2020. https://podcasts.apple.com/us/podcast/the-dream/id1435743296?i=1000462318416.
18. IBISWorld, "Vitamin & Supplement Manufacturing in the US—Market Size," 2021, https://www.ibisworld.com/industry-statistics/market-size/vita

min-supplement-manufacturing-united-states/. And Statista and Adroit Market Research, "Global Dietary Supplements Market 2018-2028," 2021, https://www.statista.com/statistics/1263458/global-dietary-supplements-market/.

19. Ann Anderson, *Snake Oil, Hustlers and Hambones: The American Medicine Show* (McFarland & Company, 2000).

20. "Quack Cures and Self-Remedies: Patent Medicine," Digital Public Library of America, accessed June 15, 2021, https://dp.la/exhibitions/patent-medicine/women-health-household-hints/?item=1304.

21. Samuel Hopkins Adams, "The Great American Fraud," accessed July 26, 2021, https://www.gutenberg.org/files/44325/44325-h/44325-h.htm.

22. John P Swann, "The 1906 Food and Drugs Act and Its Enforcement," *FDA History—Part I U.S. Food and Drug Administration*, April 10, 2013.

23. Taylor C. Wallace et al., *Dietary Supplement Regulation in the United States*, SpringerBriefs in Food, Health, and Nutrition (Springer International Publishing, 2013), https://doi.org/10.1007/978-3-319-01502-6.

24. Malcolm Gladwell, "Vitamin Makers, FDA Renewing Long Battle," *The Washington Post*, February 7, 1988, https://www.washingtonpost.com/archive/business/1988/02/07/vitamin-makers-fda-renewing-long-battle/d24b2b96-a4cf-44e8-b3a8-17c5c7f010b3/.

25. Gladwell, 1988.

26. Rahul Parikh, "Why Does Your Doctor Hate Alternative Medicine?," *Salon*, May 2, 2011, https://www.salon.com/2011/05/02/alternative_medicine_and_doctors_oz/.

27. U.S. Department of Health & Human Services, National Institutes of Health, "The NIH Almanac," https://www.nih.gov/about-nih/what-we-do/nih-almanac/national-center-complementary-integrative-health-nccih.

28. Michael Hiltzik, "Column: Orrin Hatch Is Leaving the Senate, but His Deadliest Law Will Live On," *Los Angeles Times*, January 5, 2018, https://www.latimes.com/business/hiltzik/la-fi-hiltzik-hatch-20180105-story.html.

29. U.S. Department of Health & Human Services, National Institutes of Health, Office of Dietary Supplements, https://ods.od.nih.gov/About/DSHEA_Wording.aspx; Annette Dickinson, "History and Overview of DSHEA," *Fitoterapia* 82, no. 1 (January 2011), 5–10.

30. "Supplements and Safety," *Frontline*, PBS, January 19, 2016, https://www.pbs.org/wgbh/frontline/documentary/supplements-and-safety/ (at 21:24–21:40); for the full ad: https://www.youtube.com/watch?v=_F_ZZvdHqPM.

31. "(Un)Well: Ayahuasca" (Netflix, 2020), https://www.netflix.com/title/81044208.

32. Netflix, 2020. And Carlos Suárez Álvarez, "Why You Will Never Get a Traditional Ayahuasca Treatment," Chacruna.net, 2017, https://chacruna.net/you-will-never-get-traditional-ayahuasca-treatment/.

33. Though the terms are often used interchangeably, not all consider ayahuasca and yagé to be synonymous.

34. Riccardo Vitale and Miguel Evanjuanoy Chindoy, "When Cultural Appropriation Becomes Cultural Extermination," Chacruna Institute Webinar (Chacruna Institute, November 11, 2020), https://www.crowd cast.io/e/cultural-extermination/register.

35. Carlos Suárez Álvarez, "Why You Will Never Get a Traditional Ayahuasca Treatment," Chacruna.net, 2017, https://chacruna.net/you-will-never -get-traditional-ayahuasca-treatment/.

36. Tabea Casique Coronado et al., "Declaration About Cultural Appropriation from the Spiritual Authorities, Representatives and Indigenous Organizations of the Amazon Region," UMIYAC.org, 2019, https://umi yac.org/2019/11/01/declaration-about-cultural-appropriation-from -the-spiritual-authorities-representatives-and-indigenous-organizations -of-the-amazon-region/?lang=en.

37. Kylie Cheung, "'Nine Perfect Strangers' and the Orientalist Displays of the Western Wellness Industry," *Salon.Com*, August 22, 2021, https:// www.salon.com/2021/08/22/nine-perfect-strangers-orientalism-well ness-hulu/.

38. Susanna Barkataki, *Embrace Yoga's Roots: Courageous Ways to Deepen Your Yoga Practice* (Orlando, FL: Ignite Yoga and Wellness Institute, 2020).

39. Sabrina Strings, Irene Headen, and Breauna Spencer, "Yoga as a Technology of Femininity: Disciplining White Women, Disappearing People of Color in Yoga Journal," *Fat Studies* 8, no. 3 (September 2, 2019): 334– 48, https://doi.org/10.1080/21604851.2019.1583527.

40. Ruth Flynn, "An Orientalist Orthorexia," *PopAnth*, March 4, 2020, https://popanth.com/article/an-orientalist-orthorexia-how-the-west -tokenizes-eastern-principles-of-nutrition.

41. K.K. Aggarwal and V.N. Sharma, "Anti Quackery," Indian Medical Association, accessed September 30, 2021, https://www.ima-india.org/ima /free-way-page.php?pid=143.

42. Kimberly J. Lau, *New Age Capitalism: Making Money East of Eden* (University of Pennsylvania Press, 2000), https://www.jstor.org/stable/j.ctt18crxw6.

### Chapter 3: Determinants

1. Christen Rachul et al., "COVID-19 and 'Immune Boosting' on the Internet: A Content Analysis of Google Search Results.," *BMJ Open* 10, no. 10 (2020): e040989, https://doi.org/10.1136/bmjopen-2020-040989.

2. Ed Cara, "Shady Stem Cell Clinics Are Peddling 'Immune-Boosting' Covid-19 Treatments," *Gizmodo*, May 11, 2020, https://gizmodo.com /shady-stem-cell-clinics-are-peddling-immune-boosting-co-1843348842.

3. Ralph Manuel, "12 Best Immune Booster Vitamins & Supplements For COVID-19 And Flu," *Medical Daily*, July 10, 2021, https://www.msn.com /en-us/health/medical/12-best-immune-booster-vitamins-and-supple ments-for-covid-19-and-flu/ar-AALYU1q.12 Best Immune Booster Vitamins & Supplements For COVID-19 And Flu (medicaldaily.com).

4. Sarah Garone, "A Nutritionist Shares Her 5 Favorite Immunity-Boosting Recipes to Stay Healthy during Covid-19," *CNBC Make It*, August 28,

2020, https://www.cnbc.com/2020/08/28/boost-immmune-system-with-healthy-food-and-recipes-during-covid-19-says-nutritionist.html..

5. See S M Phelan et al., "Impact of Weight Bias and Stigma on Quality of Care and Outcomes for Patients with Obesity," *Obesity Reviews* 16, no. 4 (April 2015): 319–26, https://doi.org/10.1111/obr.12266. And Elizabeth A Pascoe and Laura Smart Richman, "Perceived Discrimination and Health: A Meta-Analytic Review.," *Psychological Bulletin* 135, no. 4 (July 2009): 531–54, https://doi.org/10.1037/a0016059. And Gayla Margolin et al., "Violence Exposure in Multiple Interpersonal Domains: Cumulative and Differential Effects.," *The Journal of Adolescent Health : Official Publication of the Society for Adolescent Medicine* 47, no. 2 (August 2010): 198–205, https://doi.org/10.1016/j.jadohealth.2010.01.020.

6. David R Williams and Selina A Mohammed, "Discrimination and Racial Disparities in Health: Evidence and Needed Research.," *Journal of Behavioral Medicine* 32, no. 1 (February 2009): 20–47, https://doi.org/10.1007/s10865-008-9185-0.

7. See "County Health Rankings Model," County Health Rankings & Roadmaps, 2021, https://www.countyhealthrankings.org/explore-health-rankings/measures-data-sources/county-health-rankings-model. And Carlyn M. Hood et al., "County Health Rankings: Relationships Between Determinant Factors and Health Outcomes.," *American Journal of Preventive Medicine* 50, no. 2 (February 2016): 129–35, https://doi.org/10.1016/j.amepre.2015.08.024.

8. Jessica Morley et al., "Public Health in the Information Age: Recognizing the Infosphere as a Social Determinant of Health.," *Journal of Medical Internet Research* 22, no. 8 (August 3, 2020): e19311, *https://doi.org/10.2196/19311.* And Luciano Floridi, "Ethics in the Infosphere," *The Philosophers' Magazine*, no. 16 (November 1, 2001): 18–19, https://doi.org/10.5840/tpm20011647.

9. Morley et al. 2020. And Xuewei Chen et al., "Health Literacy and Use and Trust in Health Information," Journal of Health Communication 23, no. 8 (2018): 724–34, https://www.ncbi.nlm.nih.gov/pmc/articles/PMC6295319/.

10. Kelly M Hoffman et al., "Racial Bias in Pain Assessment and Treatment Recommendations, and False Beliefs about Biological Differences between Blacks and Whites.," *Proceedings of the National Academy of Sciences of the United States of America* 113, no. 16 (April 19, 2016): 4296–4301, https://doi.org/10.1073/pnas.1516047113.

11. Jean Heller, "AP Exposes the Tuskegee Syphilis Study: The 50th Anniversary," July 25, 2022, Associated Press, https://apnews.com/article/tuskegee-study-ap-story-investigation-syphilis-53403657e77d76f52df6c2e2892788c9. Within the 2022 piece is Heller's original 1972 AP story, "Syphilis Victims in U.S. Study Went Untreated for 40 Years."

12. Yale MacMillan Center Council on African Studies, "Carolyn Roberts on Race, Health, and Medicine in Times of COVID 19," 2020, https://african.macmillan.yale.edu/news/carolyn-roberts-race-health-and-medicine-times-covid-19.

13. David F Tolin and Edna B Foa, "Sex Differences in Trauma and Posttraumatic Stress Disorder: A Quantitative Review of 25 Years of Research," 2006, https://doi.org/10.1037/0033-2909.132.6.959.
14. Patrice Peck, "Self-Care for Black Journalists," *The New York Times*, July 14, 2020, https://www.nytimes.com/2020/07/14/style/self-care/black-journalists.html.
15. American Psychiatric Association, *Diagnostic and Statistical Manual of Mental Disorders: DSM-5*. (American Psychiatric Association, 2013).
16. Resmaa Menakem, *My Grandmother's Hands: Racialized Trauma and the Pathway to Mending Our Hearts and Bodies*, United States: Central Recovery Press, LLC, 2017.
17. Victoria M E Bridgland et al., "Why the COVID-19 Pandemic Is a Traumatic Stressor.," *PloS One* 16, no. 1 (2021): e0240146, https://doi.org/10.1371/journal.pone.0240146. And Sanketh Andhavarapu et al., "Post-Traumatic Stress in Healthcare Workers during the COVID-19 Pandemic: A Systematic Review and Meta-Analysis," *Psychiatry Research* 317 (2022): 114890, https://doi.org/10.1016/J.PSYCHRES.2022.114890.
18. Bridgland et al., 2021.
19. Mark W Miller et al., "Oxidative Stress, Inflammation, and Neuroprogression in Chronic PTSD.," *Harvard Review of Psychiatry* 26, no. 2 (2018): 57–69, https://doi.org/10.1097/HRP.0000000000000167.
20. Center for Substance Abuse Treatment, "Chapter 3: Understanding the Impact of Trauma," in *Trauma-Informed Care in Behavioral Health Services* (Substance Abuse and Mental Health Services Administration (US), 2014), https://www.ncbi.nlm.nih.gov/books/NBK207191/.
21. Division of Violence Prevention National Center for Injury Prevention and Control, "Fast Facts: Preventing Adverse Childhood Experiences," cdc.gov, 2022, https://www.cdc.gov/violenceprevention/aces/fastfact.html.
22. Bridget M Kuehn, "Growing Evidence Linking Violence, Trauma to Heart Disease.," *Circulation* 139, no. 7 (February 12, 2019): 981–82, https://doi.org/10.1161/CIRCULATIONAHA.118.038907. And Shanta R Dube et al., "Cumulative Childhood Stress and Autoimmune Diseases in Adults.," *Psychosomatic Medicine* 71, no. 2 (February 2009): 243–50, https://doi.org/10.1097/PSY.0b013e3181907888.
23. Helen King, "Once Upon a Text:_Hysteria from Hippocrates," in Hysteria Beyond Freud, edited by Sander L. Gilman et al. (Berkeley: University of California Press, 1993), 3–90. And Matt Simon, "Fantastically Wrong: The Theory of the Wandering Wombs That Drove Women to Madness," *Wired*, May 7, 2014.
24. Cecilia Tasca et al., "Women and Hysteria in the History of Mental Health.," *Clinical Practice and Epidemiology in Mental Health : CP & EMH* 8 (2012): 110–19, https://doi.org/10.2174/1745017901208010110.
25. Meghan O'Rourke, *The Invisible Kingdom: Reimagining Chronic Illness* (New York: Riverhead Books, 2022).
26. Andrew S Garner et al., "Early Childhood Adversity, Toxic Stress, and the Role of the Pediatrician: Translating Developmental Science into Lifelong

Health.," *Pediatrics* 129, no. 1 (January 1, 2012): e224-31, https://doi.org /10.1542/peds.2011-2662. And Karen E. Smith and Seth D. Pollak, "Early Life Stress and Development: Potential Mechanisms for Adverse Outcomes," *Journal of Neurodevelopmental Disorders* 12, no. 1 (December 16, 2020): 34, https://doi.org/10.1186/s11689-020-09337-y.

27. Elizabeth A Bowen and Nadine Shaanta Murshid, "Trauma-Informed Social Policy: A Conceptual Framework for Policy Analysis and Advocacy.," *American Journal of Public Health* 106, no. 2 (February 2016): 223–29, https://doi.org/10.2105/AJPH.2015.302970.

28. Substance Abuse and Mental Health Services Administration, "SAMH-SA's Concept of Trauma and Guidance for a Trauma-Informed Approach," 2014, https://store.samhsa.gov/sites/default/files/d7/priv/sma14-4884.pdf.

29. Henry Otgaar et al., "The Return of the Repressed: The Persistent and Problematic Claims of Long-Forgotten Trauma.," *Perspectives on Psychological Science: A Journal of the Association for Psychological Science* 14, no. 6 (2019): 1072–95, https://doi.org/10.1177/1745691619862306.

30. Otgaar et al. 2019. And Henry Otgaar et al., "Belief in Unconscious Repressed Memory Persists.," *Perspectives on Psychological Science : A Journal of the Association for Psychological Science* 16, no. 2 (2021): 454–60, https:// doi.org/10.1177/1745691621990628.

31. Daniel Goleman, "Proof Lacking for Ritual Abuse by Satanists," *The New York Times*, October 31, 1994, https://www.nytimes.com/1994/10/31/us /proof-lacking-for-ritual-abuse-by-satanists.html.

32. Mark L. Howe and Lauren M. Knott, "The Fallibility of Memory in Judicial Processes: Lessons from the Past and Their Modern Consequences," *Memory* 23, no. 5 (2015): 633–56, https://www.ncbi.nlm.nih.gov/pmc/arti cles/PMC4409058/.

33. Jennings Brown, "The Gateway" (Gizmodo, May 30, 2018).

34. Lisa Nichols, quoted in Rhonda Byrne, *The Secret* (Atria Books/Beyond Words, 2006).

35. The Editors of Encyclopaedia Britannica, "New Thought: Religious Movement," in *Britannica*, 1998, https://www.britannica.com/event/New -Thought. And The Editors of Encyclopaedia Britannica, "Phineas Parkhurst Quimby: American Cult Leader," in *Britannica*, 1998, https:// www.britannica.com/biography/Phineas-Parkhurst-Quimby. Also see Igor I. Sikorsky Sr. and Vincent J. Tanner Sr, Phineas Parkhurst Quimby: Maine's Godfather of New Thought (Murrells Inlet, SC: Covenant Books, 2022), and William James, The Varieties of Religious Experience: A Study in Human Nature, introduction by John E. Smith (Cambridge, MA: Harvard University Press, 1985 [1902]), especially pages 78 and following, "The Religion of Healthy-Mindedness," https://archive.org/details/varieties religi02jamegoog/page/78/mode/2up.

36. Matt Novak, "The Untold Story of Napoleon Hill, the Greatest Self-Help Scammer of All Time," *Gizmodo*, December 6, 2016, https://gizmodo.com /the-untold-story-of-napoleon-hill-the-greatest-self-he-1789385645.

37. "Manifesting—Search Term," Google Trends, 2021, https://trends.google .com/trends/explore?date=all&geo=US&q=manifesting.
38. Rebecca Jennings, "Shut Up, I'm Manifesting!," *Vox*, October 23, 2020, https://www.vox.com/the-goods/21524975/manifesting-does-it-really -work-meme.
39. Byrne, *The Secret*, 6.
40. Nitika Chopra, "Releasing Toxic Positivity and Shame.," *The Chronicles* newsletter, April 4, 2021.
41. Johanna Thompson-Hollands, Todd J Farchione, and David H Barlow, "Thought-Action Fusion across Anxiety Disorder Diagnoses: Specificity and Treatment Effects.," *The Journal of Nervous and Mental Disease* 201, no. 5 (May 2013): 407–13, https://doi.org/10.1097/NMD.0b013e31828e102c. See also B Gjelsvik et al., "Thought-Action Fusion in Individuals with a History of Recurrent Depression and Suicidal Depression: Findings from a Community Sample.," *Cognitive Therapy and Research* 42, no. 6 (2018): 782–93, https://doi.org/10.1007/s10608-018-9924-7. *(content warning for discussion of suicide.)*
42. Shayla Love, "What the Law of Attraction and These Mental Disorders Have in Common," *Vice*, April 4, 2019, https://www.vice.com/en/article/zmapne /the-idea-of-manifesting-your-future-may-be-bad-for-mental-health.
43. Marianne Williamson, *A Return to Love: Reflections on the Principles of A COURSE IN MIRACLES* (New York: Harper Perennial, 1996), 228, 240.
44. Matthew Remski, "Inside Kelly Brogan's Covid-Denying, Vax-Resistant Conspiracy Machine," *Medium*, September 15, 2020, https://gen.medium .com/inside-kelly-brogans-covid-denying-vax-resistant-conspiracy -machine-28342e6369b1.
45. Kelly Brogan, "Fear Is the Sickness," kellybroganmd.com, accessed August 2, 2022, https://www.kellybroganmd.com/blog/fear-is-the-sickness.
46. Verena Bogner, "Apparently We Can Blame Jewish Doctors for Cancer," *Vice*, March 7, 2014, https://www.vice.com/en/article/dp9gqj/germanic -new-medicine. And "Ryke Geerd Hamer und die Germanische Neue Medizin: 10. Der Approbationsentzug," https://hamer.wordpress.com/10 -der-approbationsentzug/. And Dennis Kogel, "Der wohl berühmteste deutsche 'Wunderheiler' ist tot," *Vice*, July 5, 2017, https://www.vice.com /de/article/8xagb4/der-wohl-beruhmteste-deutsche-wunderheiler-ist-tot.
47. Megan C. Hills, "Goop Contributor Kelly Brogan Peddles 'nonsense' Conspiracy Theories about Coronavirus, Cites 5G and Vaccine Companies as Real Causes," *Evening Standard*, March 25, 2020, https://www .standard.co.uk/insider/living/goop-contributor-kelly-brogan-peddles -conspiracy-theories-about-coronavirus-and-cites-5g-and-vaccine-com panies-as-causes-a4397061.html.
48. Chelsea Ritschel, "Goop Expert Says Coronavirus Doesn't Exist: 'There Is Potentially No Such Thing,'" *Independent*, March 24, 2020, https:// www.independent.co.uk/life-style/goop-coronavirus-kelly-brogan -expert-contributor-md-deaths-covid-19-a9421476.html.

49. Joanna Rothkopf, "Anti-Medication Goop Summit Expert Claims AIDS Treatment Kills and GMOs Cause Depression," *Jezebel*, December 1, 2017, https://jezebel.com/anti-medication-goop-summit-expert-claims-aids -treatmen-1820919802.

### Chapter 4: Mis- and Disinformation

1. Jennifer Saran, "Advertisers Seek Friends On Social-Networking Sites," *The Wall Street Journal*, September 3, 2004, https://www.wsj.com/articles /SB109278377163894211.

2. Jessica Morley et al., "Public Health in the Information Age: Recognizing the Infosphere as a Social Determinant of Health.," *Journal of Medical Internet Research* 22, no. 8 (August 3, 2020): e19311, https://doi.org /10.2196/19311.

3. A. Gagliardi and Alejandro R Jadad, "Examination of Instruments Used to Rate Quality of Health Information on the Internet: Chronicle of a Voyage with an Unclear Destination," *BMJ* 324, no. 7337 (March 9, 2002): 569–73, https://doi.org/10.1136/bmj.324.7337.569.

4. Morley et al., 2020.

5. Daisuke Wakabayashi, "Legal Shield for Social Media Is Targeted by Lawmakers," *New York Times*, May 28, 2020, https://www.nytimes.com /2020/05/28/business/section-230-Internet-speech.html.

6. See 47 U.S. Code § 230—Protection for private blocking and screening of offensive material, "Telecommunications," 89, https://www.govinfo .gov/content/pkg/USCODE-2020-title47/pdf/USCODE-2020-title47 -chap5-subchapII-partI-sec230.pdf. The two congressmen were Rep. Chris Cox (R-CA) and Rep. Ron Wyden (D-OR), now a senator.

7. Luke Munn, "Angry by Design: Toxic Communication and Technical Architectures," *Humanities and Social Sciences Communications* 7, no. 1 (December 30, 2020): 53, https://doi.org/10.1057/s41599-020-00550-7. And Soroush Vosoughi, Deb Roy, and Sinan Aral, "The Spread of True and False News Online.," *Science (New York, N.Y.)* 359, no. 6380 (March 9, 2018): 1146–51, https://doi.org/10.1126/science.aap9559. And William J Brady et al., "Emotion Shapes the Diffusion of Moralized Content in Social Networks.," *Proceedings of the National Academy of Sciences of the United States of America* 114, no. 28 (July 11, 2017): 7313–18, https://doi.org /10.1073/pnas.1618923114.

8. Johann Hari, *Stolen Focus: Why You Can't Pay Attention—and How to Think Deeply Again* (New York: Crown, 2022).

9. Vosoughi, Roy, and Aral, "The Spread of True and False News Online."

10. Rina Raphael, "These TikTok Creators Are Fighting Health Myths," *The New York Times*, June 29, 2022, https://www.nytimes.com/2022/06/29 /well/live/tiktok-misinformation.html?utm_source=substack&utm _medium=email.

11. Dominik Andrzej Stecula, Ozan Kuru, and Kathleen Hall Jamieson, "How Trust in Experts and Media Use Affect Acceptance of Common

Anti-Vaccination Claims," *Harvard Kennedy School Misinformation Review* 1, no. 1 (January 14, 2020), https://doi.org/10.37016/mr-2020-007.

12. Stephen R Neely et al., "Vaccine Hesitancy and Exposure to Misinformation: A Survey Analysis," 2021, https://doi.org/10.1007/s11606-021-07171-z.

13. Gordon Pennycook, Tyrone D Cannon, and David G. Rand, "Prior Exposure Increases Perceived Accuracy of Fake News," *SSRN Electronic Journal,* May 3, 2017, https://doi.org/10.2139/ssrn.2958246.

14. Zhaohui Su et al., "Mental Health Consequences of COVID-19 Media Coverage: The Need for Effective Crisis Communication Practices.," *Globalization and Health* 17, no. 1 (2021): 4, https://doi.org/10.1186/s12992-020-00654-4. And Matt Motta, Dominik Stecula, and Christina Farhart, "How Right-Leaning Media Coverage of COVID-19 Facilitated the Spread of Misinformation in the Early Stages of the Pandemic in the U.S.," *Canadian Journal of Political Science* 53, no. 2 (June 1, 2020): 335–42, https://doi.org/10.1017/S0008423920000396.

15. Matteo Pinna, Léo Picard, and Christoph Goessmann, "Cable News and COVID-19 Vaccine Uptake.," *Scientific Reports* 12, no. 1 (October 7, 2022): 16804, https://doi.org/10.1038/s41598-022-20350-0.

16. Emily Lasher et al., "COVID-19 Vaccine Hesitancy and Political Ideation among College Students in Central New York: The Influence of Differential Media Choice.," *Preventive Medicine Reports* 27 (June 2022): 101810, https://doi.org/10.1016/j.pmedr.2022.101810.

17. David Gilbert, "So Weird How Fox News Hosts Keep Defending QAnon," *Vice,* January 26, 2021, https://www.vice.com/en/article/k7akez/so-weird-how-fox-news-hosts-keep-defending-qanon. And Michael Luciano, "After Touting Ivermectin as a Covid Treatment, Fox News Hosts Ignore New Study Showing It Doesn't Work," *Mediaite,* April 7, 2022, https://www.mediaite.com/tv/fox-news-hosts-ignore-study-showing-ivermectin-doesnt-work/.

18. Will Worley, "InfoWars' Alex Jones Is a 'Performance Artist Playing a Character', Says His Lawyer," *The Independent,* April 18, 2017, https://www.independent.co.uk/news/infowars-alex-jones-performance-artist-playing-character-lawyer-conspiracy-theory-donald-trump-a7687571.html.

19. Micah Loewinger, *The Conspiracy Machine,* "Alex Jones Doesn't Care About You," *On the Media,* WNYC, June 17, 2022, https://www.wnycstudios.org/podcasts/otm/segments/alex-jones-doesnt-care-about-you-on-the-media?tab=summary.

20. Caleb Ecarma, "Fox News' Anti-Vax Mandate Messaging Is Out of Step with Its Own Strict Policies," Vanity Fair, October 7, 2021, https://www.vanityfair.com/news/2021/10/fox-news-anti-vax-messaging-policies. And Samira Sadeque, "Nearly All Fox Staffers Vaccinated for Covid Even as Hosts Cast Doubt on Vaccine," *The Guardian,* September 15, 2021, https://www.theguardian.com/media/2021/sep/15/fox-news-vaccines-testing-tucker-carlson.

21. Wall Street Journal Staff, "Facebook's Documents about Instagram and Teens, Published," *The Wall Street Journal*, September 29, 2021, https://www.wsj.com/articles/facebook-documents-instagram-teens-11632953840?mod=article_inline.

22. Written Testimony of James P. Steyer, CEO and Founder, Common Sense Media, Before the House Energy and Commerce Subcommittee on Communications and Technology Hearing on "Holding Big Tech Accountable: Targeted Reforms to Tech's Legal Immunity," December 1, 2021, https://energycommerce.house.gov/sites/democrats.energycommerce.house.gov/files/documents/Witness%20Testimony_Steyer_2021.12.01.pdf. And James P. Steyer, *Talking Back to Facebook: The Common Sense Guide to Raising Kids in the Digital Age* (New York: Scribner, 2012).

23. Iris Zhao, "Coronavirus Has Sparked Racist Attacks on Asians in Australia—Including Me," *ABC News (Australia)*, January 31, 2020, https://www.abc.net.au/news/2020-02-01/coronavirus-has-sparked-racist-attacks-on-asian-australians/11918962.

24. Associated Press, "San Francisco Lane to Be Renamed for Thai Man Killed in 2021," September 30, 2022, https://apnews.com/article/entertainment-health-covid-san-francisco-daniel-dae-kim-560dda6580081f0504b81a234d902c99.

25. Charlie Warzel, "How to Leave an Internet That's Always in Crisis," *Galaxy Brain Newsletter, The Atlantic*, July 19, 2022, https://newsletters.theatlantic.com/galaxy-brain/62d5fc32bcbd490021ad105b/quit-social-media-twitter-tiktok/.

26. Chris Hayes, "On the Internet, We're Always Famous," *The New Yorker*, September 24, 2021, https://www.newyorker.com/news/essay/on-the-Internet-were-always-famous.

27. Joan Donovan, "Trolling for Truth on Social Media," *Scientific American*, October 12, 2020, https://www.scientificamerican.com/article/trolling-for-truth-on-social-media/.

28. Wen-ying Sylvia Chou, Abby Prestin, and Stephen Kunath, "Obesity in Social Media: A Mixed Methods Analysis," *Translational Behavioral Medicine* 4, no. 3 (September 12, 2014): 314–23, https://doi.org/10.1007/s13142-014-0256-1.

29. Yongwoog Andrew Jeon et al., "Weight Stigma Goes Viral on the Internet: Systematic Assessment of YouTube Comments Attacking Overweight Men and Women.," *Interactive Journal of Medical Research* 7, no. 1 (March 20, 2018): e6, https://doi.org/10.2196/ijmr.9182.

30. Steve Kovach, "Ex-Facebook Exec Chamath Palihapitiya Says Social Media Damages Society," *Insider*, December 11, 2017, https://www.businessinsider.com/former-facebook-exec-chamath-palihapitiya-social-media-damaging-society-2017-12.

31. Jaron Lanier, *Ten Arguments for Deleting Your Social Media Accounts Right Now* (Picador, 2018).

32. Testimony of Rashad Robinson, President of Color of Change, U.S. House Committee on Energy and Commerce, Subcommittee of Com-

munications and Technology, Hearing on "Holding Big Tech Accountable: Targeted Reforms to Tech's Legal Immunity," December 1, 2021, https://energycommerce.house.gov/sites/democrats.energycommerce.house.gov/files/documents/Witness%20Testimony_Robinson_2021.12.01.pdf. And "Attachment—Additional Questions for the Record," December 1, 2021, https://docs.house.gov/meetings/IF/IF16/20211201/114268/HHRG-117-IF16-Wstate-RobinsonR-20211201-SD001.pdf.

33. Kevin Roose, "Social Media Giants Support Racial Justice. Their Products Undermine It.," *The New York Times*, June 19, 2020, https://www.nytimes.com/2020/06/19/technology/facebook-youtube-twitter-black-lives-matter.html.

34. Roose, "Social Media Giants Support Racial Justice. Their Products Undermine It."

35. Jenny Odell, *How to Do Nothing: Resisting the Attention Economy* (Melville House, 2019).

36. Odell, *How to Do Nothing*, 59.

37. Ronan Farrow, "A Pennsylvania Mother's Path to Insurrection," *The New Yorker*, February 1, 2021, https://www.newyorker.com/news/news-desk/a-pennsylvania-mothers-path-to-insurrection-capitol-riot.

38. Case No. 1:21-cr-00179-RCL, Document 67, Motion to Modify Conditions of Release, Filed May 23, 2022, https://storage.courtlistener.com/recap/gov.uscourts.dcd.228286/gov.uscourts.dcd.228286.67.0.pdf. And Joe Gorman, "Prosecutors Oppose Motion by Sandy Lake Jan. 6 Defendant," WKBN 27 (Washington, DC), June 6, 2022, https://www.wkbn.com/news/local-news/prosecutors-oppose-motion-by-sandy-lake-jan-6-defendant/. And Torsten Ove, "Judge Orders 'Pink Hat Lady' from Mercer County Confined Pending Capitol Riot Trial," *Pittsburgh Post-Gazette*, September 28, 2022, https://www.post-gazette.com/news/crime-courts/2022/09/28/pink-hat-lady-rachel-powell-capitol-riot-trial-confined-gps-western-pa-trump/stories/202209280097.

39. Alan Feuer, "Capitol Rioter Known as QAnon Shaman Pleads Guilty," *The New York Times*, September 3, 2021, https://www.nytimes.com/2021/09/03/us/politics/qanon-shaman-capitol-guilty.html.

40. Karen M. Douglas et al., "Understanding Conspiracy Theories," *Political Psychology* 40, no. S1 (February 20, 2019): 3–35, https://doi.org/10.1111/pops.12568.

41. Ali Rebeihi, "Comment Lutter Contre La Désinformation En Matière de Santé ?," *Grand Bien Vous Fasse!* podcast, March 4, 2021, https://www.franceinter.fr/emissions/grand-bien-vous-fasse/grand-bien-vous-fasse-04-mars-2021.

42. Stephan Lewandowsky and John Cook, "The Conspiracy Theory Handbook," 2020, http://sks.to/conspiracy.

43. Ricky Green and Karen M. Douglas, "Anxious Attachment and Belief in Conspiracy Theories," *Personality and Individual Differences* 125 (April 15, 2018): 30–37, https://doi.org/10.1016/J.PAID.2017.12.023.

44. Richard Fahey, "Magical Thinking: Plague, Pandemic & Unconventional Cures from the Black Death to the Covid-19," University of Notre Dame Medieval Studies Research Blog, August 21, 2020, https://sites.nd.edu/manuscript-studies/tag/conspiracy-theories/. And Nicholas Christakis, *Apollo's Arrow: The Profound and Enduring Impact of Coronavirus on the Way We Live* (New York: Little, Brown, 2020), especially chapter 5, "Us and Them."

45. PBS Newshour, "Disinformation Abounds in the Wellness Community" (PBS, February 17, 2022), https://www.pbs.org/video/in-search-of-wellness-1645137370/.

46. Janna Mandell, "Covid-19 Conspiracies Are Dividing the 'Clean' Beauty Industry," *The Lily*, March 5, 2021, https://www.thelily.com/covid-19-conspiracies-are-dividing-the-clean-beauty-industry/.

47. D. Alan Bensley et al., "The Generality of Belief in Unsubstantiated Claims," *Applied Cognitive Psychology* 34, no. 1 (January 1, 2020): 16–28, https://doi.org/10.1002/acp.3581.

48. Kiera Butler, "How Wellness Influencers Became Cheerleaders for Putin's War," *Mother Jones*, March 24, 2022, https://www.motherjones.com/politics/2022/03/how-wellness-influencers-became-cheerleaders-for-putins-war/.

49. Sam Kestenbaum, "Christiane Northrup, Once a New Age Health Guru, Now Spreads Covid Disinformation," *Washington Post*, May 3, 2022, updated May 9, 2022, https://www.washingtonpost.com/religion/2022/05/03/covid-christiane-northrup/.

50. Charlotte Ward and David Voas, "The Emergence of Conspirituality," *Journal of Contemporary Religion* 26, no. 1 (January 1, 2011): 103–21, https://doi.org/10.1080/13537903.2011.539846. See also Conspirituality 123, October 6, 2022, https://podcasts.apple.com/us/podcast/conspirituality/id1515827446?i=1000581850393 (a discussion of Ward is at 50 minutes to the end, and Voas's "give it an academic gloss" is from around 1:10:00). On her website, Ward writes of the 2011 piece: "I am the article's main author." On her approach to the use of the term "conspiracy theorist": "[P]eople don't like to be called 'conspiracy theorists'....I'm one myself (and am OK with being called that...)," https://web.archive.org/web/20150102074524/http://conspirituality.org/about/.

51. Karen M. Douglas, Robbie M. Sutton, and Aleksandra Cichocka, "The Psychology of Conspiracy Theories," *Current Directions in Psychological Science* 26, no. 6 (2017): 538–42, https://DOI: 10.1177/0963721417718261.

52. Ward and Voas.

53. Merrady Wickes, "Where Is the Line between Caution and Conspiracy?," Instagram, January 13, 2021, https://www.instagram.com/p/CJ-aRYzHzf7/. Accessed November 5, 2022.

54. N F Johnson et al., "Mainstreaming of Conspiracy Theories and Misinformation," accessed September 13, 2021, https://arxiv.org/pdf/2102.02382.pdf.

55. J Eric Oliver and Thomas Wood, "Medical Conspiracy Theories and Health Behaviors in the United States.," *JAMA Internal Medicine* 174, no. 5 (May 2014): 817–18, https://doi.org/10.1001/jamainternmed.2014.190.

56. Jen Gunter, "Worshiping the False Idols of Wellness," *The New York Times*, August 1, 2018, https://www.nytimes.com/2018/08/01/style/wellness-in dustrial-complex.html.

57. Terry Nguyen, "The Wellness World's Conspiracy Problem Is Linked to Orientalism," *Vox*, July 16, 2021, https://www.vox.com/the-goods/2257 7558/wellness-world-qanon-conspiracy-orientalism.

58. Derek Beres, Matthew Remski, and Julian Walker, "Conspirituality: 116: History Is Not a Placebo: Chinese Medicine in America (w/Tamara Venit-Shelton)," *Conspirituality Podcast*, August 11, 2022, https://podcasts .apple.com/us/podcast/conspirituality/id1515827446?i=1000575809750.

### *Chapter 5: The Anti-Vax Rabbit Hole*

1. Paul A Offit and Charlotte A Moser, "The Problem with Dr Bob's Alternative Vaccine Schedule," *Pediatrics* 123, no. 1 (January 2009): e164–69, https://doi.org/10.1542/peds.2008-2189.

2. Center for Countering Digital Hate, "The Anti-Vaxx Playbook," 2020, https://252f2edd-1c8b-49f5-9bb2-cb57bb47e4ba.filesusr.com/ugd /f4d9b9_fddbfb2a0c05461cb4bdce2892f3cad0.pdf.

3. Dean Sterling Jones, "The Gwyneth Paltrow-Approved Goop Doctor Pushing Wacky Coronavirus Conspiracies," *The Daily Beast*, March 25, 2020, https://www.thedailybeast.com/the-gwyneth-paltrow-approved-goop -doctor-pushing-wacky-coronavirus-conspiracies?ref=home.

4. Center for Countering Digital Hate, "Failure to Act," 2020, https://coun terhate.com/research/failure-to-act/.

5. Sheera Frenkel, Ben Decker, and Davey Alba, "How the 'Plandemic' Movie and Its Falsehoods Spread Widely Online," *The New York Times*, May 21, 2020, https://www.nytimes.com/2020/05/20/technology/plan demic-movie-youtube-facebook-coronavirus.html?

6. Centers for Disease Control and Prevention, *Public Health Matters* blog, "Year in Review: Measles Linked to Disneyland," December 2, 2015, https://blogs.cdc.gov/publichealthmatters/2015/12/year-in-review -measles-linked-to-disneyland/.

7. Centers for Disease Control and Prevention, "Measles History," https:// www.cdc.gov/measles/about/history.html#:~:text=Measles%20was%20 declared%20eliminated%20(absence,control%20in%20the%20Ameri cas%20region.

8. Centers for Disease Control and Prevention, "Measles Cases and Outbreaks," cdc.gov, 2021, https://www.cdc.gov/measles/cases-outbreaks.html.

9. World Health Organization, "Ten Threats to Global Health in 2019," https:// www.who.int/news-room/spotlight/ten-threats-to-global-health-in-2019.

10. Renee DiResta, "Anti-Vaxxers Are Using Twitter to Manipulate a Vaccine Bill," *WIRED*, June 8, 2015, https://www.wired.com/2015/06/antivaxx ers-influencing-legislation/.

11. Tara Haelle, "Opinion: This Is the Moment the Anti-Vaccine Movement Has Been Waiting For," *The New York Times*, August 31, 2021, https:// www.nytimes.com/2021/08/31/opinion/anti-vaccine-movement.html.

12. See, for example, Erica X Eisen, " 'The Mark of the Beast': Georgian Britain's Anti-Vaxxer Movement," *The Public Doman Review*, April 27, 2021, https://publicdomainreview.org/essay/the-mark-of-the-beast-georgian-britains-anti-vaxxer-movement.

13. Brian Deer, "How the Case Against the MMR Vaccine Was Fixed," *BMJ* 342 (January 6, 2011): c5347, https://www.bmj.com/content/342/bmj.c5347.full.

14. Jeremy Laurance, "I Was There When Wakefield Dropped His Bombshell," *The Independent*, January 29, 2010, https://www.independent.co.uk/life-style/health-and-families/health-news/i-was-there-when-wakefield-dropped-his-bombshell-1882548.html.

15. Robert T. Chen and Frank DeStefano, "Vaccine Adverse Events: Causal or Coincidental?," *The Lancet* 351, no. 9103 (February 28, 1998): 611–12, https://doi:10.1016/S0140-6736(05)78423-3.

16. Laurance, "I Was There When Wakefield Dropped His Bombshell."

17. Brian Deer, "MMR—The Truth Behind the Crisis," *London Sunday Times*, February 22, 2004. This piece and others by Deer published the same day can be accessed at https://briandeer.com/mmr/lancet-deer-2.htm.

18. Brian Deer, *The Doctor Who Fooled the World: Science, Deception, and the War on Vaccines* (Baltimore: Johns Hopkins University Press, 2020), 116–17.

19. Anna Merlan, *Republic of Lies: American Conspiracy Theorists and Their Surprising Rise to Power* (Metropolitan Books, 2019), https://www.amazon.com/dp/1250159059/ref=rdr_ext_tmb.

20. Deer, "How the Case Against the MMR Vaccine Was Fixed." The figure cited by Deer is "£435 643, plus expenses." See also Deer, *The Doctor Who Fooled the World: Science, Deception, and the War on Vaccines*.

21. Merlan, Republic of Lies, 124. And Azhar Hussain et al., "The Anti-Vaccination Movement: A Regression in Modern Medicine," Cureus 10, no. 7 (July 3, 2018): e2919, https://doi: 10.7759/cureus.2919. And Carrie Macmillan, "Herd Immunity: Will We Ever Get There?," Yale Medicine, May 21, 2921, https://www.yalemedicine.org/news/herd-immunity#:~:text=Measles%2C%20for%20example%2C%20spreads%20so,measles%20will%20no%20longer%20spread.

22. Michael Hiltzik, "Jenny McCarthy: Anti-Vaxxer, Public Menace," *Los Angeles Times*, January 27, 2015, https://www.latimes.com/business/hiltzik/la-fi-mh-jenny-mccarthy-antivaxxer-public-menace-20150127-column.html.

23. "Making Sense of Dr. Andrew Wakefield Now," Texas Children's Hospital blog, unsigned post, March 2011, https://www.texaschildrens.org/blog/2011/03/making-sense-dr-andrew-wakefield-now.

24. Timothy Buie, "The Relationship of Autism and Gluten.," *Clinical Therapeutics* 35, no. 5 (May 1, 2013): 578–83, https://doi.org/10.1016/j.clinthera.2013.04.011.

25. Iain D Croall, Nigel Hoggard, and Marios Hadjivassiliou, "Gluten and Autism Spectrum Disorder.," *Nutrients* 13, no. 2 (February 9, 2021): 572, https://doi.org/10.3390/nu13020572.

26. Jane Marie, "Drowning in the Conspira-Sea," *The Dream*, January 2020.

27. "Biographies of Steering Committee Members," Commission for Countering Extremism, blog post, November 5, 2021, gov.uk, https://extremismcommission.blog.gov.uk/2020/04/15/our-steering-committee/.

28. Imran Ahmed, "The Anti-Vaxx Playbook: Anti-Vaxxers' Digital Plan to Disrupt COVID-19 Vaccines," Center for Humane Technology Webinar, February 12, 2021.

29. Renée DiResta, "Anti-vaxxers Think This Is Their Moment," *The Atlantic*, December 20, 2020, https://www.theatlantic.com/ideas/archive/2020/12/campaign-against-vaccines-already-under-way/617443/.

30. Elizabeth Culliford and Paresh Dave, "YouTube Bans Coronavirus Vaccine Misinformation," *Reuters*, October 14, 2020, https://www.reuters.com/article/health-coronavirus-youtube-int/youtube-bans-coronavirus-vaccine-misinformation-idUSKBN26Z21R.

31. Gerrit De Vynck, "YouTube Is Banning Prominent Anti-Vaccine Activists and Blocking All Anti-Vaccine Content," *Washington Post*, September 29, 2021, https://www.washingtonpost.com/technology/2021/09/29/youtube-ban-joseph-mercola/. And Jessica Bursztynsky, "YouTube Bans High-Profile Anti-Vaccine Accounts," *CNBC*, September 29, 2021, https://www.cnbc.com/2021/09/29/youtube-bans-high-profile-anti-vaccine-accounts.html.

32. Dr. Joseph Mercola (@mercola), Twitter, September 27, 2022, https://twitter.com/mercola/status/1574745812143575040.

33. Dr. Joseph Mercola (@mercola), Twitter, September 22, 2022, https://twitter.com/mercola/status/1573032238735818754.

34. Anna Merlan, "Anti-Vaccine Organization Children's Health Defense Says It Was Banned from Instagram and Facebook," *Vice*, August 18, 2022, https://www.vice.com/en/article/ake3xz/anti-vaccine-organization-childrens-health-defense-says-it-was-banned-from-instagram-and-facebook.

35. Sirin Kale, "Chakras, Crystals and Conspiracy Theories: How the Wellness Industry Turned Its Back on Covid Science," *The Guardian*, November 11, 2021, https://www.theguardian.com/world/2021/nov/11/injecting-poison-will-never-make-you-healthy-how-the-wellness-industry-turned-its-back-on-covid-science.

36. Center for Countering Digital Hate, "Malgorithm: How Instagram's Algorithm Publishes Misinformation and Hate to Millions During a Pandemic," 2021, https://counterhate.com/research/malgorithm-fix-instagram/.

37. David A Broniatowski et al., "Weaponized Health Communication: Twitter Bots and Russian Trolls Amplify the Vaccine Debate.," *American Journal of Public Health* 108, no. 10 (October 12, 2018): 1378–84, https://doi.org/10.2105/AJPH.2018.304567.

38. Jonathan Jarry, "The Anti-Vaccine Movement in 2020," *McGill Office for Science and Society*, May 22, 2020, https://www.mcgill.ca/oss/article/covid-19-pseudoscience/anti-vaccine-movement-2020.

39. R. J. Reinhart, "Fewer in U.S. Continue to See Vaccines as Important," Gallup, January 14, 2020, https://news.gallup.com/poll/276929/fewer -continue-vaccines-important.aspx.

40. Andrea Michelson, "White Republicans Are More Likely to Reject the COVID-19 Vaccine," *Insider,* March 15, 2021, https://www.businessinsider .com/white-republicans-more-likely-to-reject-covid-19-vaccine-2021-3.

41. National Institutes of Health, "NCI Study Highlights Pandemic's Dispro-portionate Impact on Black, American Indian/Alaska Native, and Latino Adults," October 4, 2021, https://www.nih.gov/news-events/news-releases /nci-study-highlights-pandemics-disproportionate-impact-black-ameri can-indian-alaska-native-latino-adults.

42. Brandy Zadrozny and Char Adams, "Covid's Devastation of Black Com-munity Used as 'Marketing' in New Anti-Vaccine Film," *NBC News,* March 11, 2021, https://www.nbcnews.com/news/nbcblk/covid-s-devastation -black-community-used-marketing-new-anti-vaxxer-n1260724.

43. Victoria Milko, "Concern among Muslims over Halal Status of COVID-19 Vaccine," *ABC News,* December 20, 2020, https://abcnews.go.com /Health/wireStory/concern-muslims-halal-status-covid-19-vaccine -74826269.

44. Briony Swire-Thompson and David Lazer, "Public Health and Online Misinformation: Challenges and Recommendations," *Annual Review of Public Health* 41, no. 1 (April 2, 2020): 433–51, https://doi.org/10.1146 /annurev-publhealth-040119-094127.

45. Ariana Eunjung Cha, "False Claims Tying Coronavirus Vaccines to Infer-tility Drive Doubts among Women of Childbearing Age," *The Washington Post,* February 22, 2021, https://www.washingtonpost.com/health/2021 /02/22/women-vaccine-infertility-disinformation/.

46. World Health Organization, "Coronavirus Disease (COVID-19): Preg-nancy, Childbirth and the Postnatal Period," March 15, 2022, https:// www.who.int/news-room/questions-and-answers/item/coronavirus-dis ease-covid-19-pregnancy-and-childbirth.

47. Brandy Zadrozny and Aliza Nadi, "How Anti-Vaxxers Target Grieving Moms and Turn Them into Crusaders against Vaccines," *NBC News,* Sep-tember 24, 2019, https://www.nbcnews.com/tech/social-media/how-anti -vaxxers-target-grieving-moms-turn-them-crusaders-n1057566.

48. Anita Emly, "Our Natural Lifestyle Didn't Prevent Flu," *Voices for Vaccines* blog, October 26, 2020, https://www.voicesforvaccines.org/natural-life style-didnt-prevent-flu/.

49. Lewandowsky and Cook, "The Conspiracy Theory Handbook."

50. Rachael Piltch-Loeb et al., "Testing the Efficacy of Attitudinal Inocula-tion Videos to Enhance COVID-19 Vaccine Acceptance: Quasi-Experimental Intervention Trial.," *JMIR Public Health and Surveillance* 8, no. 6 (June 20, 2022): e34615, https://doi.org/10.2196/34615.

51. Dell Cameron, "A Lawsuit Against Instagram Could Find a Way Around Section 230," *Gizmodo,* June 9, 2022, https://gizmodo.com/instagram -facebook-papers-meta-teen-spence-lawsuit-sect-1849036765.

52. Marc-André Argentino, "Conspiracy Pilled: The Growing Public Health Threat Posed by Conspiracy Theories and Disinformation," *Concordia. Ca*, December 22, 2020, https://www.concordia.ca/cunews/offices/vprgs /sgs/public-scholars-20/2020/12/22/conspiracy-pilled.html.

53. DiResta, "Anti-vaxxers Think This Is Their Moment."

54. Katie Cloyd, "She Went Viral for Her Antivaxx Stance—Now She's Asking Folks to Get Their COVID Vaccine," *Scary Mommy*, February 4, 2021, updated February 6, 2021, https://www.scarymommy.com/measles-cos tume-mom-get-covid-vaccine.

55. Robert Crawford, "Healthism and the Medicalization of Everyday Life," *International Journal of Health Services* 10, no. 3 (July 1980): 365–88, https://doi.org/10.2190/3H2H-3XJN-3KAY-G9NY.

## Chapter 6: Dubious Diagnoses and Spurious Cures

1. See J Bradford Rice et al., "Long-Term Systemic Corticosteroid Exposure: A Systematic Literature Review.," *Clinical Therapeutics* 39, no. 11 (November 1, 2017): 2216–29, https://doi.org/10.1016/j.clinthera.2017.09 .011. And Jessica L Hwang and Roy E Weiss, "Steroid-Induced Diabetes: A Clinical and Molecular Approach to Understanding and Treatment.," *Diabetes/Metabolism Research and Reviews* 30, no. 2 (February 2014): 96– 102, https://doi.org/10.1002/dmrr.2486.

2. Halis Kaan Akturk et al., "Over-the-Counter 'Adrenal Support' Supplements Contain Thyroid and Steroid-Based Adrenal Hormones.," *Mayo Clinic Proceedings* 93, no. 3 (2018): 284–90, https://doi.org/10.1016/j .mayocp.2017.10.019.

3. Caldwell Esselstyn, "Dr. Esselstyn's Prevent & Reserve Heart Disease Program," http://www.dresselstyn.com/site/books/prevent-reverse/about-the -book/. And Caldwell Esselstyn, *Prevent and Reverse Heart Disease: The Revolutionary, Scientifically Proven, Nutrition-Based Cure* (New York: Avery /Penguin, 2008), 38 ("Every mouthful of oils and animal products, including dairy products, initiates an assault…a cascade of free radicals in our bodies"), 68, 118, 120, 123.

4. Rip Esselstyn, "We Are PLANTSTRONG," https://plantstrong.com /about/.

5. O'Rourke, *The Invisible Kingdom*, 4, 130.

6. Pew Research Center, "2. Americans' Health Care Behaviors and Use of Conventional and Alternative Medicine," 2017, https://www.pewresearch .org/science/2017/02/02/americans-health-care-behaviors-and -use-of-conventional-and-alternative-medicine/.

7. Ted J Kaptchuk et al., "Components of Placebo Effect: Randomised Controlled Trial in Patients with Irritable Bowel Syndrome.," *BMJ (Clinical Research Ed.)* 336, no. 7651 (May 3, 2008): 999–1003, https://doi.org /10.1136/bmj.39524.439618.25.

8. Brian Resnick, "The Weird Power of the Placebo Effect, Explained," *Vox*, July 7, 2017, https://www.vox.com/science-and-health/2017/7/7/15792188 /placebo-effect-explained.

9. Luana Colloca and Fabrizio Benedetti, "Placebo Analgesia Induced by Social Observational Learning.," *Pain* 144, no. 1–2 (July 2009): 28–34, https://doi.org/10.1016/j.pain.2009.01.033.

10. Harrison, *Anti-Diet*, 106–8. See also Peter R Gibson, Gry I Skodje, and Knut E A Lundin, "Non-Coeliac Gluten Sensitivity," *Journal of Gastroenterology and Hepatology* 32 (March 2017): 86–89, https://doi.org/10.1111/jgh.13705.

11. John M. Kelley, "Lumping and Splitting: Toward a Taxonomy of Placebo and Related Effects," *International Review of Neurobiology* 139 (January 1, 2018): 29–48, https://doi.org/10.1016/BS.IRN.2018.07.011.

12. National Institutes of Health, "Complementary and Alternative Medicine Funding by NIH Institute/Center," accessed June 22, 2022, https://www.nccih.nih.gov/about/budget/complementary-and-alternative-medicine-funding-by-nih-institutecenter.

13. Paul A. Offit, "Studying Complementary and Alternative Therapies," *JAMA* 307, no. 17 (May 2, 2012): 1803–4, https://doi.org/10.1001/jama.2012.518.

14. National Institutes of Health, "Research Portfolio Online Reporting Tools (RePORT)," 2022, https://reporter.nih.gov/search.

15. James L. Wilson, *Adrenal Fatigue: The 21st Century Stress Syndrome* (Petaluma, CA: Smart Publications, 2001), 61.

16. Wilson, *Adrenal Fatigue*, 6.

17. Doctor Wilson's Original Formulations. 2020. "Save 10% off Adrenal Fatigue: The 21st Century Stress Syndrome." Facebook, September 16, 2020. https://www.facebook.com/doctorwilsonsoriginalformulations/posts/3177574762341128. And AdrenalFatigue.org. "About James L. Wilson." https://adrenalfatigue.org/about-james-l-wilson-dc-nd-phd/ (Accessed July 28, 2021; now deleted).

18. Cedars-Sinai Staff, "Debunking Adrenal Fatigue," *Cedars-Sinai Blog*, January 16, 2018, https://www.cedars-sinai.org/blog/debunking-adrenal-fatigue.html.

19. Flavio A Cadegiani and Claudio E Kater, "Adrenal Fatigue Does Not Exist: A Systematic Review.," *BMC Endocrine Disorders* 16, no. 1 (August 24, 2016): 48, https://doi.org/10.1186/s12902-016-0128-4.

20. Endocrine Society, "Adrenal Fatigue | Endocrine Society," Endocrine.org, January 25, 2022, https://www.endocrine.org/patient-engagement/endocrine-library/adrenal-fatigue. Accessed November 8, 2022.

21. James L. Wilson, "Adrenal Fatigue Questionnaire," icahealth.com, 2019, https://icahealth.com/wp-content/uploads/Adrenal-Fatigue-Questionnaire-FINAL.pdf.

22. Cadegiani and Kater, 2016.

23. Cadegiani and Kater, 2016.

24. Endocrine Society, 2022.

25. Agnieszka Pazderska and Simon Hs Pearce, "Adrenal Insufficiency — Recognition and Management.," *Clinical Medicine (London, England)* 17, no. 3 (June 2017): 258–62, https://doi.org/10.7861/clinmedicine.17-3-258.

26. Sonia Ratib et al., "Long-Term Topical Corticosteroid Use and Risk of Skin Cancer: A Systematic Review.," *JBI Database of Systematic Reviews and Implementation Reports* 16, no. 6 (June 2018): 1387–97, https://doi.org/10.11124/JBISRIR-2017-003393.

27. Nutrition Forum, "Briefs: Stuart Berger Attacked," *Nutrition Forum*, March 1990. https://www.scribd.com/document/386045636/Nutrition-Forum.

28. U.S. Department of Health and Human Services Office on Women's Health, "Vaginal Yeast Infections," womenshealth.gov, 2021, https://www.womenshealth.gov/a-z-topics/vaginal-yeast-infections.

29. Heather L. Paladine and Urmi A. Desai, "Vaginitis: Diagnosis and Treatment," *American Family Physician* 97, no. 5 (March 1, 2018): 321–29, https://www.aafp.org/afp/2018/0301/p321.html.

30. See Laura Buggio et al., "Probiotics and Vaginal Microecology: Fact or Fancy?," *BMC Women's Health* 19, no. 1 (2019): 25, https://doi.org/10.1186/s12905-019-0723-4. And Jhhm van de Wijgert and M C Verwijs, "Lactobacilli-Containing Vaginal Probiotics to Cure or Prevent Bacterial or Fungal Vaginal Dysbiosis: A Systematic Review and Recommendations for Future Trial Designs.," *BJOG : An International Journal of Obstetrics and Gynaecology* 127, no. 2 (2020): 287–99, https://doi.org/10.1111/1471-0528.15870.

31. Genetic and Rare Diseases Information Center, "Systemic Candidiasis," National Institutes of Health website, accessed August 9, 2021, https://rarediseases.info.nih.gov/diseases/1076/systemic-candidiasis.

32. Jan Kullberg and Maiken C. Arendrup, "Invasive Candidiasis," *New England Journal of Medicine* 373 (2015): 1445–46. And Centers for Disease Control and Prevention, "Invasive Candidiasis Statistics," cdc.gov, 2021, https://www.cdc.gov/fungal/diseases/candidiasis/invasive/statistics.html.

33. Executive Committee of the American Academy of Allergy and Immunology, "Position Statement: Candidiasis Hypersensitivity Syndrome," *Journal of Allergy and Clinical Immunology* 78, no. 2 (1986), https://www.jacionline.org/article/S0091-6749(86)80073-2/pdf.

34. Lubna Mohammed et al., "The Interplay Between Sugar and Yeast Infections: Do Diabetics Have a Greater Predisposition to Develop Oral and Vulvovaginal Candidiasis?," *Cureus* 13, no. 2 (February 18, 2021), https://doi.org/10.7759/cureus.13407.

35. Sophia Ehrström, Anna Yu, and Eva Rylander, "Glucose in Vaginal Secretions Before and After Oral Glucose Tolerance Testing in Women with and without Recurrent Vulvovaginal Candidiasis," *Obstetrics & Gynecology* 108, no. 6 (December 2006): 1432–37, https://doi.org/10.1097/01.AOG.0000246800.38892.fc.

36. M Weig et al., "Limited Effect of Refined Carbohydrate Dietary Supplementation on Colonization of the Gastrointestinal Tract of Healthy Subjects by Candida Albicans.," *The American Journal of Clinical Nutrition* 69, no. 6 (June 1999): 1170–73, https://doi.org/10.1093/ajcn/69.6.1170.

37. Svitrigaile Grinceviciene et al., "Non-Response to Fluconazole Maintenance Treatment (ReCiDiF Regimen) for Recurrent Vulvovaginal Candidosis Is

Not Related to Impaired Glucose Metabolism.," *Mycoses* 60, no. 8 (August 2017): 546–51, https://doi.org/10.1111/myc.12626.

38. Mark Hyman, "About Functional Medicine," drhyman.com, accessed June 5, 2022, https://drhyman.com/about-functional-medicine/.

39. National Organization for Rare Disorders (NORD), "Desmoid Tumor," NORD Rare Disease Database, accessed November 17, 2021, https://rarediseases.org/rare-diseases/desmoid-tumor/.

40. Oriana M. Damas, Luis Garces, and Maria T. Abreu, "Diet as Adjunctive Treatment for Inflammatory Bowel Disease: Review and Update of the Latest Literature," *Current Treatment Options in Gastroenterology* 17, no. 2 (June 9, 2019): 313–25, https://doi.org/10.1007/s11938-019-00231-8.

41. Meghan O'Rourke, *The Invisible Kingdom: Reimagining Chronic Illness* (New York: Riverhead Books, 2022).

### Chapter 7: Scams, Schemes, and Snake Oil

1. Beau Donelly and Nick Toscano, "Backlash over App Developer Belle Gibson's Missing Charity Money," *The Sydney Morning Herald*, March 9, 2015, https://www.smh.com.au/technology/backlash-over-app-developer -belle-gibsons-missing-charity-money-20150309-13yzd4.html.

2. Beau Donelly and Nick Toscano, *The Woman Who Fooled the World: Belle Gibson's Cancer Con, and the Darkness at the Heart of the Wellness Industry* (London: Scribe, 2017).

3. Belle Gibson, Instagram, March 31, 2014. https://web.archive.org/web /20140331040756/http://instagram.com/healing_belle.

4. Donelly and Toscano, *The Woman Who Fooled the World*, 53, 62–62, 120, 162.

5. Beau Donelly and Nick Toscano, "Charity Money Promised by 'Inspirational' Health App Developer Belle Gibson Not Handed Over," *The Age*, March 15, 2015, https://www.theage.com.au/technology/charity-money -promised-by-inspirational-health-app-developer-belle-gibson-not -handed-over-20150306-13xgqk.html.

6. Clair Weaver, "My Lifelong Struggle with the Truth," *Australian Women's Weekly*, May 2015. https://www.nowtolove.co.nz/news/real-life/belle-gib son-my-lifelong-struggle-with-the-truth-6860.

7. Federal Court of Australia, *Director of Consumer Affairs Victoria v. Gibson*, FCA 240, March 15, 2017, https://www.judgments.fedcourt.gov.au/judg ments/Judgments/fca/single/2017/2017fca0240.

8. Clark Stanley, *The Life and Adventures of the American Cow-Boy: Life in the Far West*, 1897, https://archive.org/details/F596S822CowboyImages/page /n45/mode/2up.

9. Brooks McNamara, *Step Right Up*, Revised (University Press of Mississippi, 1996), https://www.google.com/books/edition/Step_right_up/LZw VhxaljA8C?hl=en&gbpv=1&bsq=kickapoo.

10. Brooks McNamara, "The Indian Medicine Show," *Educational Theatre Journal* 23, no. 4 (December 1971): 431, https://doi.org/10.2307/320 5750.

11. Lakshmi Gandhi, "A History Of 'Snake Oil Salesmen,'" *Code Switch* (NPR, August 26, 2013), https://www.npr.org/sections/codeswitch/2013/08/26/215761377/a-history-of-snake-oil-salesmen.
12. United States Bureau of Chemistry, "4944. Misbranding of 'Clark Stanley's Snake Oil Liniment.,'" in *Service and Regulatory Announcements, Issues 21-30* (U.S. Government Printing Office, 1917), 592, https://books.google.com/books?id=-Og7AAAAYAAJ&q=%22snake+oil%22&pg=PA592#v=snippet&q=%22snake%20oil%22&f=false.
13. American Society of Clinical Oncology, "ASCO 2020 National Cancer Opinions Survey," October 2020, https://www.asco.org/sites/new-www.asco.org/files/content-files/2020-ASCO-National-Cancer-Opinions-Survey-All-Findings.pdf.
14. Scotty Hendricks, "Is Postmodernism Really Anti-Science?," *Big Think*, October 15, 2018, https://bigthink.com/the-present/is-postmodernism-really-anti-science/. And Ava Kofman, "Bruno Latour, the Post-Truth Philosopher, Mounts a Defense of Science," *The New York Times Magazine*, October 25, 2018, https://www.nytimes.com/2018/10/25/magazine/bruno-latour-post-truth-philosopher-science.html. And Brian Duignan, "Postmodernism," in *Encyclopedia Britannica*, September 4, 2020, https://www.britannica.com/topic/postmodernism-philosophy.
15. Jeffrey Jones, "Confidence in U.S. Institutions Down; Average at New Low," *Gallup*, July 5, 2022, https://news.gallup.com/poll/394283/confidence-institutions-down-average-new-low.aspx.
16. Sharon LaFraniere and Noah Weiland, "Walensky, Citing Botched Pandemic Response, Calls for C.D.C. Reorganization," *The New York Times*, August 17, 2022, https://www.nytimes.com/2022/08/17/us/politics/cdc-rochelle-walensky-covid.html?smid=nytcore-ios-share&referringSource=articleShare.
17. Bill Whitaker, "Did the FDA Ignite the Opioid Epidemic? — 60 Minutes" (CBS News, 2019), https://www.cbsnews.com/news/opioid-epidemic-did-the-fda-ignite-the-crisis-60-minutes/. And U.S. General Accounting Office, "GAO-04-110, Prescription Drugs: OxyContin Abuse and Diversion and Efforts to Address the Problem," gao.gov, 2004, https://www.gao.gov/assets/a240885.html.
18. Whitaker, 2019.
19. Will Stone and Pien Huang, "CDC Issues New Opioid Prescribing Guidance, Giving Doctors More Leeway to Treat Pain," *National Public Radio*, November 3, 2022.
20. Tressie McMillan Cottom, "Opinion: We're All 'Experts' Now. That's Not a Good Thing.," *The New York Times*, January 10, 2022, https://www.nytimes.com/2022/01/10/opinion/scams-were-all-experts.html.
21. Xiao Xiao, Xiangyi Li, and Yi Zhou, "Financial Literacy Overconfidence and Investment Fraud Victimization," *Economics Letters* 212 (March 1, 2022): 110308, https://doi.org/10.1016/J.ECONLET.2022.110308.
22. Charlie Warzel, "Opinion: Don't Go Down the Rabbit Hole," *The New York Times*, February 18, 2021, https://www.nytimes.com/2021/02/18

/opinion/fake-news-media-attention.html. And Mike Caulfield, "SIFT (The Four Moves)," *Hapgood*, June 19, 2019, https://hapgood.us/2019/06 /19/sift-the-four-moves/.

23. Michael Caulfield, "Recalibrating Our Approach to Misinformation," *EdSurge News*, December 19, 2018, https://www.edsurge.com/news/2018 -12-19-recalibrating-our-approach-to-misinformation.

24. Warzel, 2021.

25. Nicole Einbinder, "The History of Young Living's Gary Young and His 'Essential Oils' Empire," *Business Insider*, July 29, 2020, https://www.busi nessinsider.com/young-living-gary-young-founder-essential-oils-2020-7.

26. Various, 1983, https://assets.documentcloud.org/documents/6940096 /Essential-Oils-Combined.pdf.

27. Various, 1983, https://assets.documentcloud.org/documents/6940096 /Essential-Oils-Combined.pdf.

28. John Hurst, "'Patient' Submits Blood (From Cat), Is Given Diagnosis," *Los Angeles Times*, October 23, 1987. https://www.latimes.com/archives /la-xpm-1987-10-23-mn-10747-story.html.

29. Herb Greenberg, "Multi-Level Marketing Critic: Beware 'Main Street Bubble,'" *CNBC*, January 9, 2013, https://www.cnbc.com/id/100366687.

30. Jon M Taylor, "The Case (for and) against Multi-Level Marketing," Chapter 7, 2011, https://www.ftc.gov/sites/default/files/documents/public _comments/trade-regulation-rule-disclosure-requirements-and-prohibi tions-concerning-business-opportunities-ftc.r511993-00008%C2%A0 /00008-57281.pdf.

31. World Federation of Direct Selling Associations, "2020/2021 Annual Report," 2021.

32. Direct Selling Association, "Direct Selling in the United States: 2021 Industry Overview," 2022, https://www.dsa.org/statistics-insights.

33. Claudia Gross and Dirk Vriens, "The Role of the Distributor Network in the Persistence of Legal and Ethical Problems of Multi-Level Marketing Companies," *Journal of Business Ethics* 156 (May 12, 2017), https://doi.org /10.1007/s10551-017-3556-9.

34. Abby Ohlheiser, "FDA Warns Three Companies Against Marketing Their Products as Ebola Treatments or Cures," *Washington Post*, September 24, 2014, https://www.washingtonpost.com/news/to-your-health/wp /2014/09/24/fda-warns-three-companies-against-marketing-their-prod ucts-as-ebola-treatments-or-cures/.

35. Nicole Einbinder, "Some Members of Multilevel-Marketing Company Young Living Are Making Questionable Claims about 'Essential Oils' Curing Cancer and Coronavirus," *Insider*, July 29, 2020, https://www .businessinsider.com/young-living-essential-oils-medical-claims -2020-7?r=US&IR=T.

36. Rachel Monroe, "How Essential Oils Became the Cure for Our Age of Anxiety," *The New Yorker*, October 2, 2017, https://www.newyorker.com /magazine/2017/10/09/how-essential-oils-became-the-cure-for-our -age-of-anxiety.

37. Zenab Aly Torky et al., "Chemical Profiling, Antiviral and Antiproliferative Activities of the Essential Oil of Phlomis Aurea Decne Grown in Egypt.," *Food & Function*, April 29, 2021, https://doi.org/10.1039/d0fo03417g.

38. Mahmoud M Suhail et al., "Boswellia Sacra Essential Oil Induces Tumor Cell-Specific Apoptosis and Suppresses Tumor Aggressiveness in Cultured Human Breast Cancer Cells.," *BMC Complementary and Alternative Medicine* 11 (December 15, 2011): 129, https://doi.org/10.1186/1472-6882-11-129.

39. Federal Trade Commission Staff to Mark A. Wolfert, doTERRA general counsel, April 24, 2020, https://truthinadvertising.org/wp-content/uploads/2020/12/2020-FTC-MLM-COVID-Warning-Letters.pdf.

40. Steven A. Burd, "How Safeway Is Cutting Health-Care Costs," *Wall Street Journal*, June 12, 2009, https://www.wsj.com/articles/SB12447680402630 8603.

41. David S. Hilzenrath, "Misleading Claims about Safeway Wellness Incentives Shape Health-Care Bill," *The Washington Post*, January 17, 2010, https://www.washingtonpost.com/wp-dyn/content/article/2010/01/15/AR2010011503319.html.

42. Quoted in Hilzenrath, "Misleading Claims about Safeway Wellness Incentives Shape Health-Care Bill."

43. Barack Obama, "Remarks by the President to the Annual Conference of the American Medical Association," June 15, 2009, https://obamawhitehouse.archives.gov/the-press-office/remarks-president-annual-conference-american-medical-association.

44. Carrie Dennett, "Are Workplace Wellness Programs All They're Cracked up to Be? Here's the Deal," *The Seattle Times*, October 4, 2021, https://www.seattletimes.com/life/wellness/are-workplace-wellness-programs-all-theyre-cracked-up-to-be-heres-the-deal/.

45. Damon Jones, David Molitor, and Julian Reif, "What Do Workplace Wellness Programs Do? Evidence from the Illinois Workplace Wellness Study.," *The Quarterly Journal of Economics* 134, no. 4 (November 2019): 1747–91, https://doi.org/10.1093/qje/qjz023.

46. Kaiser Family Foundation, "2021 Employer Health Benefits Survey: Summary of Findings," November 10, 2021, https://www.kff.org/report-section/ehbs-2021-summary-of-findings/.

47. Ravi Telugunta, Komal Urde, and Onkar Sumant, "Workplace Wellness Market Size, Share & Industry Analysis 2027," Allied Market Research, 2020, https://www.alliedmarketresearch.com/workplace-wellness-market.

48. Jones, Molitor, and Reif, 2019.

49. Zirui Song and Katherine Baicker, "Effect of a Workplace Wellness Program on Employee Health and Economic Outcomes," *JAMA* 321, no. 15 (April 16, 2019): 1491, https://doi.org/10.1001/jama.2019.3307.

50. Zirui Song and Katherine Baicker, "Health and Economic Outcomes Up to Three Years after a Workplace Wellness Program: A Randomized Controlled Trial," *Health Affairs* 40, no. 6 (June 1, 2021): 951–60, https://doi.org/10.1377/hlthaff.2020.01808.

51. Charlotte Lieberman, "What Wellness Programs Don't Do for Workers," *Harvard Business Review*, August 14, 2019, https://hbr.org/2019/08/what-wellness-programs-dont-do-for-workers.

**Chapter 8: From Wellness to Well-Being**

1. Crawford, "Healthism and the Medicalization of Everyday Life," 376, 379.

2. Quoted in Crawford, "Healthism and the Medicalization of Everyday Life," 375, 379.

3. Kathie Obradovich, "Des Moines University Will Train Medical Students to Manage Mental Health," *Des Moines Register*, October 30, 2017, https://www.desmoinesregister.com/story/opinion/columnists/kathie-obradovich/2017/10/30/des-moines-university-joins-nami-mental-health-training/812645001/.

4. Jon Favreau, "Offline: Dr. Vivek Murthy on Defeating Doomscrolling with Human Connection," *Pod Save America*, December 12, 2021, https://podcasts.apple.com/us/podcast/pod-save-america/id1192761536?i=1000544700439.

5. Statement of Frances Haugen, United States Senate Committee on Commerce, Science, and Transportation, Subcommittee on Consumer Protection, Product Safety, and Data Security, October 4, 2021, https://www.commerce.senate.gov/services/files/FC8A558E-824E-4914-BEDB-3A7B1190BD49.

6. *McDougal v. Fox News Network, LLC*, No. 1:2019cv11161—Document 39 (SDNY 2020), https://law.justia.com/cases/federal/district-courts/new-york/nysdce/1:2019cv11161/527808/39/.

7. Chris Fox, "Social Media: How Might It Be Regulated?," *BBC News*, November 12, 2020, https://www.bbc.com/news/technology-54901083.

8. Tim De Chant, "Algorithms Shouldn't Be Protected by Section 230, Facebook Whistleblower Tells Senate," *Ars Technica*, October 6, 2021, https://arstechnica.com/tech-policy/2021/10/algorithms-shouldnt-be-protected-by-section-230-facebook-whistleblower-tells-senate/.

9. Renee DiResta, "Free Speech Is Not the Same as Free Reach," *WIRED*, August 30, 2018, https://www.wired.com/story/free-speech-is-not-the-same-as-free-reach/.

10. Imran Ahmed, U.S. Congress House of Representatives Energy & Commerce Committee, Subcommittee on Consumer Protection & Commerce Hearing on Holding Big Tech Accountable: Legislation to Build a Safer Internet, December 9, 2021, https://www.youtube.com/watch?v=TmYN2grMMp8 (at 2:15:23–2:16:18).

11. Nathalie Maréchal, spoken testimony, U.S. Congress House of Representatives Energy & Commerce Committee, Subcommittee on Consumer Protection & Commerce Hearing on Holding Big Tech Accountable: Legislation to Build a Safer Internet, December 9, 2021, https://www.youtube.com/watch?v=TmYN2grMMp8 (at 2:03:00–2:03:54).

12.  Forum on Information & Democracy, "Working Group on Infodemics Policy Framework," 2020, https://informationdemocracy.org/wp-content /uploads/2020/11/ForumID_Report-on-infodemics_101120.pdf.

13.  Thomas C. O'Brien, Ryan Palmer, and Dolores Albarracin, "Misplaced Trust: When Trust in Science Fosters Belief in Pseudoscience and the Benefits of Critical Evaluation," *Journal of Experimental Social Psychology* 96 (September 1, 2021): 104184, https://doi.org/10.1016/J.JESP.2021.104184.

14.  Caroline Wilbert, "Dark Chocolate Prevents Heart Disease," *WebMD*, September 25, 2008, https://www.webmd.com/heart-disease/news/2008 0925/dark-chocolate-prevents-heart-disease. Accessed August 24, 2022.

15.  Dennis Thompson, "That Morning Cup of Coffee May Extend Your Life," *U.S. News & World Report*, May 31, 2022. Accessed August 24, 2022.

16.  Clement Adebamowo et al., "High School Dietary Dairy Intake and Teen-age Acne," *Journal of the American Academy of Dermatology* 52, no. 2 (2005). Note that a number of other studies have *not* found such an association— an example of how contradictory findings between studies are fairly common in nutritional epidemiology. Given the current state of the science, the official position of the American Academy of Dermatology is that "no specific dietary changes are recommended in the management of acne."

17.  Christie Aschwanden, "You Can't Trust What You Read about Nutrition," *FiveThirtyEight*, January 6, 2016, https://fivethirtyeight.com/features /you-cant-trust-what-you-read-about-nutrition/.

18.  Mayo Clinic Staff, "Cancer Risk: What the Numbers Mean," mayoclinic .org, February 17, 2022, https://www.mayoclinic.org/diseases-conditions /cancer/in-depth/cancer/art-20044092.

19.  Cal Newport, *Digital Minimalism: Choosing a Focused Life in a Noisy World* (Portfolio/Penguin, 2019).

20.  Sebene Selassie, "Wellness is Not Worth," *The Call for Connection Newsletter*, December 4, 2021.

21.  Julianne Holt-Lunstad, "Why Social Relationships Are Important for Physical Health: A Systems Approach to Understanding and Modifying Risk and Protection.," *Annual Review of Psychology* 69 (2018): 437–58, https://doi.org/10.1146/annurev-psych-122216-011902.

22.  Eric S Kim, Victor J Strecher, and Carol D Ryff, "Purpose in Life and Use of Preventive Health Care Services.," *Proceedings of the National Academy of Sciences of the United States of America* 111, no. 46 (November 18, 2014): 16331–36, https://doi.org/10.1073/pnas.1414826111.

23.  Eric S Kim et al., "Sense of Purpose in Life and Subsequent Physical, Behavioral, and Psychosocial Health: An Outcome-Wide Approach.," *American Journal of Health Promotion: AJHP* 36, no. 1 (January 2022): 137– 47, https://doi.org/10.1177/08901171211038545.

24.  See Lisa Payne et al., "Improving Well-Being after Traumatic Brain Injury through Volunteering: A Randomized Controlled Trial.," *Brain Injury* 34, no. 6 (2020): 697–707, https://doi.org/10.1080/02699052.2020

.1752937. And Laura A Weiss et al., "The Long and Winding Road to Happiness: A Randomized Controlled Trial and Cost-Effectiveness Analysis of a Positive Psychology Intervention for Lonely People with Health Problems and a Low Socio-Economic Status.," *Health and Quality of Life Outcomes* 18, no. 1 (June 2, 2020): 162, https://doi.org/10.1186/s12955 -020-01416-x.

# Index

# ABOUT THE AUTHOR

**Christy Harrison,** MPH, RD, is a registered dietitian nutritionist, certified intuitive eating counselor, and journalist who has been covering food and health for more than twenty years. She is the author of *Anti-Diet* and the producer and host of the podcasts Food Psych and Rethinking Wellness, which have helped tens of thousands of people around the world think critically about diet and wellness culture and develop more peaceful relationships with food. Her writing has appeared in the *New York Times, SELF,* BuzzFeed, WIRED, Refinery29, *Gourmet, Slate,* the Food Network, and many other publications, and her work is regularly featured in national print and broadcast media.